Working in Care Settings

Common Induction Standards

Val Michie

2nd Edition

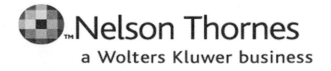
Nelson Thornes
a Wolters Kluwer business

Text © Val Michie 2007

Illustrations © Nelson Thornes Ltd 2007

First published in 2004

Second edition published in 2007 by:
Nelson Thornes Ltd
Delta Place
27 Bath Road
CHELTENHAM
GL53 7TH
United Kingdom

07 08 09 10 11 / 10 9 8 7 6 5 4 3 2 1

A catalogue record for this book is available from the British Library

ISBN 978 0 7487 8158 4

Illustrations by Clinton Banbury and Angela Lumley

Page make-up by Florence Productions Ltd, Stoodleigh, Devon

Printed in Slovenia by Korotan

Contents

Introduction

Why read this book?

Everyone who starts to work in care or who changes their caring role or work setting must receive induction training to a certain standard. Skills for Care has developed a set of Common Induction Standards (CIS), which are intended to be met within a 12-week induction period and which will enable care workers to give high quality care and support, provide recognition for their work, and prepare them for entry onto NVQ health and social care programmes.

The reading material in this book covers the knowledge and understanding that you need to complete your induction training:

- Chapter 1 aims to develop your knowledge and understanding of the principles of care
- Chapter 2 aims to develop your knowledge and understanding of your job role and the organisation you work for
- Chapter 3 aims to develop your knowledge and understanding of the health and safety legislation that applies to care work and how you should put it into practice
- Chapter 4 aims to develop your knowledge and understanding of communication techniques and how you can use them to encourage others to communicate with you
- Chapter 5 aims to develop your knowledge and understanding of abuse and neglect and how to respond when you think they may be taking place
- Chapter 6 aims to help you know and understand how you can develop in your role as a worker.

The reading material also provides much of the underpinning knowledge and understanding needed for the Health and Social Care

NVQ units at level 2. These are highlighted at the beginning of each chapter. In addition, completing the activities gives you the chance to develop your discussion, reading and writing skills and to build your portfolio for the key skill qualification Communication at level 1.

How to achieve the Common Induction Standards

This book has been written in a style and at a level that will appeal to you if you have not had recent experience of learning or if you are not confident in your ability to learn.

The activities throughout the book are linked to the Skills for Care Common Induction Standards and give you the opportunity to think about, check and demonstrate your knowledge and understanding.

Case studies focus what you are learning into a practical situation that you may experience at work. They help you to imagine what you would do if you were involved in the issue being presented.

What do you think? encourages you to reflect on what you have just read, or to think about the way you work.

Develop good work practice invites you to concentrate on your workplace, looking at procedures and the way you work with the people you support and your colleagues. Can these be improved?

Check your understanding is a way for you to make sure that you have understood the topics you have just read.

Completing the activities will provide the evidence you need to achieve the Standards.

The book has been written primarily to support care workers who work with older people. However, it also provides much of the knowledge and understanding needed if you work with adults and young people who have disabilities and learning difficulties.

I hope you enjoy this book and that it helps you find achievement, fulfilment and success in your job. I also hope that it whets your appetite for further learning and self-development.

MAPPING GRID

Mapping of chapters and activities to the Skills for Care Common Induction Standards, Health and Social Care NVQ level 2 units and key skill Communication at level 1

Chapter and links to HSC level 2 units	Activity	Links to Common Induction Standards	Links to key skill Communication at level 1
1. Understand the	1	1.1.1	C1.2
principles of care	2	1.1.2	C1.2
HSC 21, 22, 23, 24	3	1.1.3	C1.2
	4	1.2.1	C1.2
	5	1.2.2	C1.2
	6	1.2.3	C1.2
	7	1.3.1	C1.2
	8	1.3.2	C1.1, C1.2
	9	1.3.3	C1.2
	10	1.3.4	C1.1, C1.2
	11	1.3.5	C1.1, C1.2
	12	1.4.1	C1.1, C1.2
	13	1.4.2	C1.1, C1.2
	14	1.4.3	C1.1, C1.2, C1.3
2. Understand the	15	2.1.1	C1.2, C1.3
organisation and the	16	2.1.2	C1.1, C1.2
role of the worker	17	2.1.3	C1.1, C1.2, C1.3
HSC 21, 22, 23, 24	18	2.1.4	C1.1, C1.2
	19	2.2.1	C1.2
	20	2.2.2	C1.2, C1.3
	21	2.3.1	C1.2
	22	2.3.2	C1.1, C1.2
3. Maintain safety at	23	3.1.1	C1.2, C1.3
work	24	3.1.2	C1.1, C1.2, C1.3
HSC 21, 22, 23, 24	25	3.1.3	C1.2, C1.3
	26	3.1.4	C1.2

	27	3.2.1	C1.2
	28	3.2.2	C1.2
	29	3.2.3	C1.1
	30	3.2.4	C1.1, C1.2
	31	3.3.1	C1.1
	32	3.4.1	C1.1, C1.2
	33	3.4.2, 3.4.3	C1.1, C1.2
	34	3.5.1	C1.1, C1.2, C1.3
	35	3.5.2	C1.1, C1.2, C1.3
	36	3.5.3	C1.1, C1.2
	37	3.6.1	C1.1
	38	3.6.2	C1.1, C1.2
	39	3.6.3	C1.1
	40	3.7.1	C1.1, C1.2, C1.3
	41	3.7.2	C1.1, C1.2
4. Communicate effectively HSC 21, 22, 24	42	4.1.1	C1.1, C1.2
	43	4.1.2	C1.1, C1.2, C1.3
	44	4.1.3	C1.2
	45	4.2.1	C1.1, C1.2
	46	4.2.2	C1.1, C1.2
	47	4.2.3, 4.2.4	C1.2, C1.3
	48	4.3.1	C1.2
	49	4.3.2	C1.1, C1.2
	50	4.3.3	C1.1, C1.2, C1.3
	51	4.3.4	C1.1, C1.2, C1.3
5. Recognise and respond to abuse and neglect HSC 24	52	5.1.1	C1.1, C1.2
	53	5.1.2, 5.1.3	C1.1, C1.2
	54	5.2.1	C1.2
	55	5.3.1	C1.2
	56	5.4.1, 5.4.2	C1.1, C1.2, C1.3
	57	5.4.3	C1.2
	58	5.5.1	C1.2
	59	5.5.2	C1.1, C1.2
	60	5.5.3	C1.2
	61	5.5.4	C1.2

Understand the principles of care

The principles of care set the standards for how you should work with people who need care or support, their families and friends, your colleagues, and people from other organisations. This chapter aims to develop your knowledge and understanding of the principles of care so that you can develop work practices that support the care, safety and well being of the <u>individuals</u> you work with.

Successful completion of the activities in this chapter will allow you to demonstrate your understanding of the Common Induction Standard *Understand the principles of care*. It will also give you an opportunity to produce evidence for the key skills unit Communication at level 1.

What is covered in this chapter?

This chapter contributes to the knowledge and understanding you need for the following NVQ Care units at level 2:
HSC 21 : Communicate with, and complete records for individuals
HSC 22 : Support the health and safety of yourself and individuals
HSC 23 : Develop your knowledge and practice
HSC 24 : Ensure your own actions support the care, protection and well being of individuals

1.1 THE VALUES

The <u>care values</u> are the beliefs that underpin care work. Using the care values in your work is good practice because it shows the people you support that you value them. The following sections describe how you can use the care values in your work.

1.1.1 Understand the need to promote the following care values at all times

Respect

Respecting the people you support demonstrates that you value them for who they are. It shows that you have consideration for their values, beliefs, likes and dislikes. It also means letting their preferences shape the way you work with them. Respect runs through all of the care values.

Individuality

Each of us has a unique set of genes and life experiences that set us apart from everybody else. Although we have much in common with each other, even the closest friends and family members have different personalities, opinions and ways of doing things. Also, our <u>diverse</u> cultural backgrounds mean that we have different customs, values and beliefs.

Recognising people's individuality in the way you support them demonstrates that you value them. By treating people as individuals you will help them feel good about themselves and reassured that you understand them.

Rights

Except in very special circumstances, everybody has rights.

Denying people their rights makes them feel that they don't count, that they are worthless. Respecting people's rights in the way you support them shows them that you value them. It makes them feel important and well-regarded.

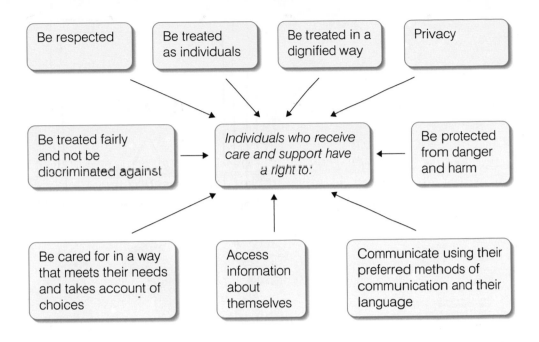

Privacy

We all have a right to privacy, for example in matters of personal information and correspondence, financial affairs, telephone calls, relationships and maintaining personal hygiene. Except in exceptional circumstances, no-one should interfere with what we want to be kept private. If someone intrudes into private lives we lose trust in them.

Respecting people's right to privacy in the way you support them shows that you value them. For example, respect the closed door – it could mean that a private meeting or telephone conversation is taking place, that someone is using the toilet or is having a bath. A letter, bank statement or pension book is private unless you have been given permission to read it; and two people locked in quiet conversation means a private discussion may be taking place and you may not be welcome to join in.

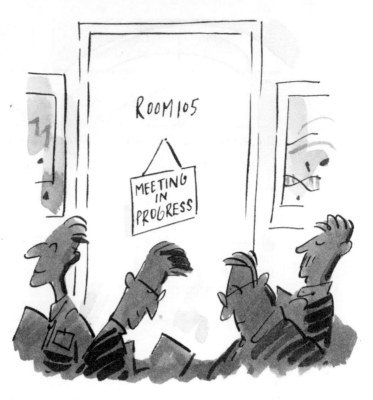

It is important to respect other people's privacy

Independence

Becoming independent is a normal part of human development. Staying as independent as possible is important because it means being able to do what we want, when we want. It means being responsible for ourselves, staying in control, living the life we want to live, being confident and having a feeling of self-worth.

Helping people to stay independent in the way you support them shows that you value them. It means respecting what independence they already have and encouraging them to be as responsible for themselves as they can, for example in managing their money, in dealing with their relationships, in getting around and in maintaining their personal hygiene and appearance.

Choice

We all need to be able to make choices for ourselves. Making choices helps us to be independent and in control of our lives. Not being able to make choices can be frustrating and make us dependent on others.

Encouraging the people you support to make choices and respecting the choices they make, for example about how they are cared for, shows that you value them and want them to remain independent and in charge of their own lives.

Dignity

Dignity is about self-respect and being proud of ourselves. We feel dignified when, for example, we behave, dress or do our job in ways that we feel are right and proper and that we are comfortable with. If our dignity is taken away, we can feel cheapened, ashamed and degraded, and we lose our pride in ourselves.

Respecting people's dignity in the way that you support them shows that you value them. If someone has a preference for a way of doing things or presenting themselves to others, you should respect that preference and not force your ways and ideas onto them. You should always help others to feel proud of themselves.

Partnership

Care work is not about working *for* people in need of care and support. Instead, it involves working in partnership *with* them. Partnership working demonstrates that you value people as individuals and have respect for their knowledge, experience and rights. It demonstrates that you value the choices they make and have respect for what they can and cannot do for themselves.

What do you think?

ACTIVITY 1

Use the table below to show how and why you must use the care values in your work.

Care values	How I use the values in my work	Why I must use the values in my work
Respect		
Individuality		
Rights		
Privacy		
Independence		
Choice		
Dignity		
Partnership		

1.1.2 Understand the need to promote equal opportunities for the individual(s) you are supporting

How do you feel about the following statements?

- the amputee in ward 5
- wheelchair users
- the elderly.

The problem with these expressions is that they describe people according to just one of their characteristics. We call this labelling. Labelling has the effect of making people feel that their other characteristics and qualities have no value.

It is human nature to judge people according to characteristics associated with their appearance and the way they behave. Stereotyping is when we assume that everyone who shares one or two characteristics is the same in every other way. But while one older person may be confused, it is far from the truth that all older people are confused. Stereotyping, like labelling, doesn't value people's individuality.

It is also human nature to pre-judge people before we know them properly. Prejudices are the ideas and beliefs we have about the people we pre-judge. They are usually negative and are based on people's age, sex, appearance (e.g. size and skin colour), disability, job, social class, religion and politics. Prejudices are generally unfounded and untrue.

The way you label and stereotype people and your negative prejudices must never be allowed to influence the way you support people. If, for example, you are prejudiced against someone because of the colour of their skin, their age or their religion and you show your thoughts in the way you talk or act, you will be behaving in a discriminatory way.

Discrimination means treating a person unfairly because of the way they have been labelled, stereotyped or pre-judged. Examples of discrimination include:

- not asking older people for their opinion because they are considered to be 'past it', despite their wisdom and understanding

- treating someone who is physically disabled as dim-witted, even though it may only be their legs that don't work.

Unfair treatment also takes place because of a lack of understanding of the difficulties some people face, for example:

- people with learning difficulties or mental health problems are often treated with suspicion because they don't behave in an expected way
- steps, stairs and doors discriminate against people who have <u>mobility problems</u>
- information in written English discriminates against people who have difficulty seeing or using the English language
- spoken information, fire alarms, etc. discriminate against people who have hearing problems
- menus that don't provide a variety of foods discriminate against people who have special dietary needs
- staff who are either all women or all men discriminate against people whose religion requires them to be cared for by a member of the same sex.

Being discriminated against makes people feel worthless, frustrated and angry. The British Government has passed a number of laws that protect our right to fair treatment and freedom from discrimination.

These laws also ensure that we each have the same access to the same life chances as everyone else, for example education, employment and services. This is what is meant by <u>equal opportunities</u>.

Some people need help to access life chances. For example, people who have a <u>sensory impairment</u>, are disabled, old, or who have learning difficulties or health problems may need help to study, do their job and use health and social care services. For this reason, equal opportunities requires that help is put in place to make sure that no-one is disadvantaged or treated less fairly than everyone else.

<u>Care service providers</u> use anti-discrimination laws to write procedures that describe how <u>care workers</u> will meet people's care and support needs. The <u>General Social Care Council's</u> <u>Code of Practice</u> for care

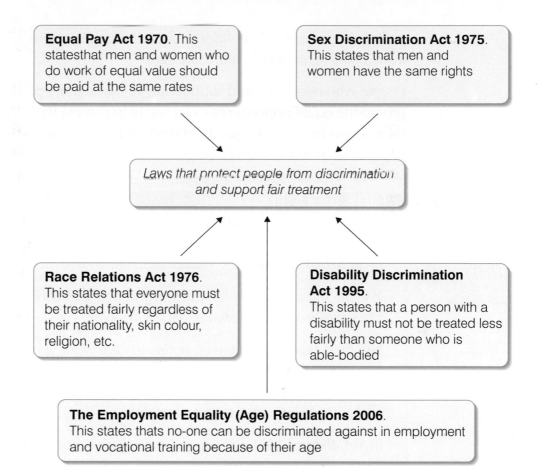

Equal Pay Act 1970. This statesthat men and women who do work of equal value should be paid at the same rates

Sex Discrimination Act 1975. This states that men and women have the same rights

Laws that protect people from discrimination and support fair treatment

Race Relations Act 1976. This states that everyone must be treated fairly regardless of their nationality, skin colour, religion, etc.

Disability Discrimination Act 1995. This states that a person with a disability must not be treated less fairly than someone who is able-bodied

The Employment Equality (Age) Regulations 2006. This states thats no-one can be discriminated against in employment and vocational training because of their age

workers also describes their responsibilities and the standards they are expected to meet when carrying out their work. By following procedures and the GSCC Code of Practice, care workers can be confident that their work promotes equal opportunities, and that they treat everyone fairly and according to their individual needs, regardless of their age, sex, colour, ability, religion and so on.

Do you follow anti-discriminatory procedures and the Code of Practice? Do you make sure that no-one in your care is disadvantaged? Admitting that your work practice can be less than perfect on occasion will help you to challenge your behaviour and improve the way you give care and support. It will also put you in a better position to recognise and challenge other people's unfair behaviour. If you hear someone using offensive or hurtful language or see evidence of unfair behaviour, challenge them politely. If you are not confident about doing this on your own, get help from a colleague or your line manager.

People who need care and support are vulnerable. By playing your part in promoting equal opportunities you will help protect their rights, promote their access to fair and equal treatment and, by making them feel valued, improve their sense of well being.

CHECK YOUR UNDERSTANDING

1.1.2

ACTIVITY 2

CASE STUDY: *Lazy Days*

Wayne, Ingrid and Ken have recently joined the workforce at Lazy Days Residential Care Home for older people.

You have heard Wayne, who is new to care work, grumbling at having to work with 'wrinklies' and 'psychos' and with residents who need help to use the toilet. He also 'has a problem' with immigrants and with people who don't hear or see very well.

Ingrid, the new deputy manager, has cut down on staffing, in particular during the afternoons when recreational activities take place.

Ken, the chef, has bought new kitchen equipment. This means he has less money to spend on food so is no longer offering any choice on the menu. He is currently storing his new equipment in the lift and in one of the downstairs toilets.

How will Wayne, Ingrid and Ken's behaviour affect equal opportunities for the residents at Lazy Days?

Why is it important that people who need support have access to equal opportunities?

How do you promote equal opportunities for the people you support?

▲▲

1.1.3 Understand the need to support and respect diversity and different cultures and values

Diversity is to do with the differences between people. For example, people from different cultures live differently. They also have different attitudes, expectations, values, religious beliefs, traditions and customs, which they hold dear and pass down from one generation to the next.

Other important differences between people include their:

- **Ethnic background** People from different ethnic backgrounds have, for example, a different religion, language and physical appearance
- **Social class** People's social class depends on what they earn, their occupation, how much education they have had and where they live
- **Gender** Gender is to do with femininity and masculinity. Different people have different ideas about what makes a person feminine and masculine
- **Age** Society is populated by people of different ages, e.g. children, youths, young adults, adults, middle-aged people and older people. Each age group has its own set of experiences

- **Family structure** There are many different family structures in the world, including <u>nuclear families</u>, <u>extended families</u>, <u>one-parent families</u>, <u>same sex parent families</u>, <u>reconstituted families</u> and <u>single-person households</u>
- **Disability** Many people have a disabling physical or mental health condition, or have a physical disability
- **Religious and <u>secular beliefs</u>** Beliefs are ideas that we believe in and think of as true. People living in Britain hold a wide range of religious and secular beliefs, and they include atheists, Buddhists, Christians, Hindus, Humanists, Jehovah's Witnesses, Jews, Muslims, Pagans, Rastafarians and Sikhs.

Caring for and supporting a diverse range of people will give you the chance to improve your understanding of different ways of life and to understand how and why people communicate, behave and dress as they do. It will also give you an opportunity to:

- learn from their experiences. Different people have a wealth of experiences that they will be delighted to share with you if you show an interest. Listening to what they tell you will improve your knowledge and help you see things from different perspectives
- improve their sense of well being. Getting to know and understand a diverse range of people helps promote tolerance and mutual respect. As a result, communication improves, relationships grow and people's sense of well being develops
- show that you value them and have respect for their attitudes, beliefs and values. We all have the right to think what we want, believe what we want and to practise our religion or beliefs in the way that we choose
- learn new ways of doing things. Supporting people who do things differently from you will help you develop skills and techniques as well as improve your current performance.

People who need care and support are different in many ways. By supporting and respecting their many differences, you will make them feel valued, promote their rights, and grow and develop both personally and in your work.

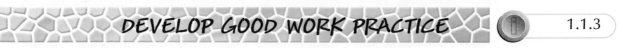

DEVELOP GOOD WORK PRACTICE 　　1.1.3

ACTIVITY 3

Make a note below to describe three ways in which you support and respect diversity and different cultures and values:

1

2

3

Now describe three ways in which you can improve the way you work with regard to supporting and respecting diversity:

1

2

3

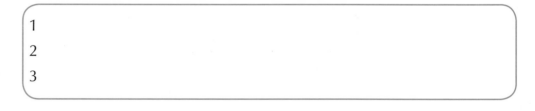

1.2 CONFIDENTIALITY

1.2.1 Understand the importance of confidentiality

<u>Confidentiality</u> is to do with respecting privacy and being discreet.

Respecting privacy is one of the care values. As you read earlier, except in special circumstances, everybody has a right to have their privacy respected, both in their personal lives and in their affairs with other people and organisations. Being discreet means being careful about the kind of information you pass on and who you pass it on to.

In order to carry out your role as a care worker, you need to know a great deal of personal and sensitive information about the people you support.

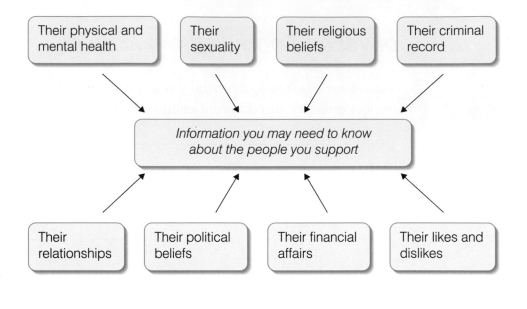

Their physical and mental health	Their sexuality	Their religious beliefs	Their criminal record

Information you may need to know about the people you support

Their relationships	Their political beliefs	Their financial affairs	Their likes and dislikes

CASE STUDY: Ivor

Ivor had a nervous breakdown in his fifties which led to him becoming homeless, abusing drugs and spending a period of time in prison. He is now 73 and living in a residential care home.

How do you think Ivor would feel if this information became a subject of gossip where he lives? He might feel rejected by the other residents, and become lonely and isolated. He might feel betrayed and would think twice before telling anybody anything about himself in the future. However, his care workers need to have information about him in order to meet his needs.

As a care worker you have a responsibility to safeguard all the information that people tell you. Except in certain situations that you will read about shortly, you must never repeat what you are told to anybody else unless:

- they need the information to do their job, e.g. your colleagues and visiting health and social care professionals
- the person concerned has given you permission. Family and friends may make enquiries but you must not give them information without

permission. It may be that the person doesn't want anyone to know why or how they are receiving care.

If you receive a telephone enquiry about someone you support, you must not disclose any information unless you:

- recognise the caller's voice
- have confirmed their identity – you could ask for their phone number, check it out and ring them back
- have permission to give them the information they are asking for.

If a visitor arrives asking for information, before you let them in you should:

- confirm their identity – they may have an official ID card or a photo driving licence
- confirm with your line manager that they have a right to visit
- check with the person concerned that they wish to see the visitor.

Your organisation's procedures describe who you can share information with and under what circumstances. You will be asked to look at these shortly. If you are given permission to pass information on to someone else, make sure that nobody can overhear your conversation. Respect people's privacy by having discussions behind closed doors.

Personal and sensitive information is written into records such as:

- care plans and case notes
- medical records
- Medicines Administration Records
- observation charts.

The Data Protection Act 1998 is in place to make sure that personal and sensitive information is protected. It states that records must be stored so that the details within them remain confidential. Your organisation obeys the Data Protection Act by having procedures that describe how records are to be protected.

Protecting someone's records shows respect for their right to privacy. It also prevents them from being harmed through the misuse of their personal information. You have a responsibility to maintain the confidentiality of records by not allowing other people to read them unless:

- they have been given permission by the person concerned
- they need to know the information.

Your organisation's procedures describe who you can share recorded information with and under what circumstances. You will be asked to look at these procedures shortly.

You can help maintain the confidentiality of records by making sure that nobody can oversee what you write. If you are using a computer, make sure that the monitor is angled so that others can't see what you are typing. Finally, look after records carefully – don't leave them lying around, put them away as soon as you've finished with them; and store them securely in locked filing cabinets or in computer files that can only be opened by people with a secure password.

By demonstrating your ability to respect privacy and be discreet, you will demonstrate that you are trustworthy and that you apply the principles of care in your work.

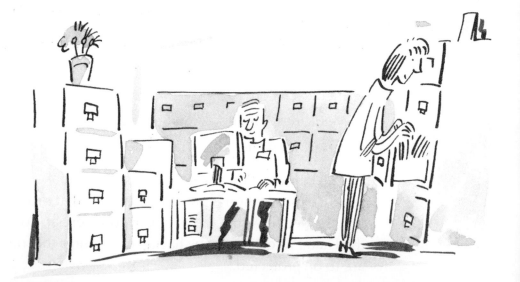

Records and reports should be stored appropriately in order to protect your service users' confidentiality

What do you think?

ACTIVITY 4

1 Think about your attitude to maintaining confidentiality. Do you respect people's privacy? Are you discreet at all times? Be honest! If not, how do you think your behaviour affects the people you support? Do you think they trust you and tell you all that you need to know?

2 Make some notes on why is it necessary for care workers to maintain confidentiality.

1.2.2 Understand the limits of confidentiality

There may be occasions when you need to 'break' confidentiality. What this means is that 'need-to-know' information about someone you support can be passed on without their permission. However, except in exceptional circumstances, they must be told exactly what information has been passed on (disclosed) as soon as possible.

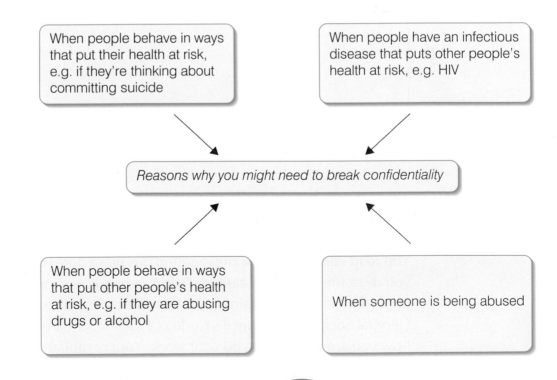

When people behave in ways that put their health at risk, e.g. if they're thinking about committing suicide

When people have an infectious disease that puts other people's health at risk, e.g. HIV

Reasons why you might need to break confidentiality

When people behave in ways that put other people's health at risk, e.g. if they are abusing drugs or alcohol

When someone is being abused

Because you may need to break confidentiality, you must never promise someone to keep a secret before you hear what they have to say. If you feel that you need to pass on what they tell you, reassure them that you are doing so in their best interests and that you will only tell the people who are there to help. Be tactful, diplomatic and sensitive to their feelings and the situation. They need to know that your judgement is sound and considered.

CHECK YOUR UNDERSTANDING

1.2.2

ACTIVITY 6

1 Make a list of occasions when you would need to 'break' confidentiality, with reasons.

2 How would you explain your action to the person concerned?

1.2.3 Know how to apply your organisation's policies and procedures about sharing information

You read earlier that your organisation has procedures describing how you must meet people's care and support needs, e.g. promoting equal opportunities and maintaining confidentiality. You also read that the General Social Care Council's Code of Practice for care workers describes how you are expected to do your work. Your organisation also has procedures that let you know what information you can share with others and with whom you can share it.

You have a responsibility to know and use your organisation's procedures. The next activity gives you an opportunity to find out about procedures relating to the sharing of information and to think about how you apply them in your work.

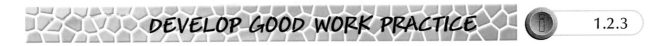

DEVELOP GOOD WORK PRACTICE   1.2.3

ACTIVITY 7

Read your organisation's procedures on sharing information to enable you to complete the following table.

Information I can share	Who I can share the information with

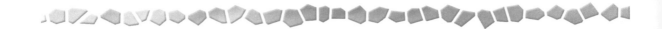

1.3   PERSON CENTRED APPROACHES

Care workers need to have a person centred approach in their work with people who need support. A person centred approach is based on the principles of care and involves:

- respecting the privacy and dignity of the people you work with
- letting the preferences, wishes and needs of the people you work with shape the way you support them

- making sure that the way you work with them is based around them and not you or the organisation you work for
- encouraging them to make <u>informed choices</u> about their care so that they can remain in control of their own lives.

1.3.1 Know how to support the privacy and dignity of the individual(s) you support

The previous section described how to maintain the privacy of personal, sensitive information. This section looks at how you can demonstrate respect for people's privacy by preventing unwanted intrusion into their lives. It also looks at how you can help maintain their dignity or self-respect.

How can you show respect for the privacy and dignity of the people you support?

Show consideration for their 'personal space'. This is the private space they have around them and which no-one should enter unless they have permission. Different people have different ideas of what makes for personal space. Some people enjoy being close together while others prefer to maintain their distance, especially from people they are not emotionally close to. Invading people's personal space without being invited shows a lack of respect and can make them feel threatened and insecure.

Make sure that there is a quiet, private area where their conversations cannot be overheard. Telephone conversations, chats with family and friends and discussions with professionals about health and care needs are very personal and not intended to be made public. Careless talk and gossip by care workers and the people they support, about conversations they overheard and which are meant to be private, make life very unpleasant for the people concerned.

Make sure that doors to personal areas such as bedrooms and bathrooms can indicate when the room is being used. It can be very embarrassing if someone enters a room when the occupant is, for example, using the toilet or changing their clothes or continence pad. Always knock before entering a room, and, if appropriate, wait for an answer.

Behave in such a way that you make them feel they matter. For example, be interested, kind and complimentary and have a positive attitude. In particular, don't complain about how busy you are or interrupt your work with them to talk to other people or answer the telephone. This is not only rude, it also makes the person you are working with feel that they are unimportant and of no concern. If you must take a telephone call or respond to another situation, ask for their permission and tell them that you will be back as quickly as you can. This will help them feel that they are your main concern and preserve their self-esteem.

Safeguard their modesty and self-respect at all times. For example, protect them from embarrassment – if they are undressed, using a bedpan or being washed or examined, shut the door, use blankets or screens as shields, and make sure that curtains and blinds are closed. Also, check how they would like to be addressed. Some people are happy to be called by their first (given) name; others prefer to be addressed by their family name, e.g. Mr Smith, Mrs Khan, Dr Gibson.

Make sure they are able to present themselves to the world as they would like. Many people are very particular about their image and are uncomfortable if their clothes, hair and so on are dirty, messy or smelly. Make sure that they are fresh and hygienic; that they have their own freshly laundered and ironed clothes to wear; that they are shaved as often as they wish; that there hair is in a style that pleases them; and that any soiled clothes are changed straightaway. Many people are also very particular about the personality they present to the world. Be alert to situations which, for example, shy and retiring people find difficult and protect them from being hurt, upset or offended.

DEVELOP GOOD WORK PRACTICE

1.3.1

ACTIVITY 7

1 Make a list of situations when the privacy and dignity of the people you support might be invaded.

2 Describe the methods you currently use to protect their privacy and dignity.

3 Explain how you can improve your work practice to make sure that you never allow their privacy and dignity to be invaded.

1.3.2 Understand the importance of finding out the history, preferences, wishes and needs of the people you are supporting

You read earlier that we each have a unique set of genes and different life experiences or histories. The sorts of experiences that make you an individual include those to do with:

- **Your family** The only child, the eldest or youngest, and the child from a single-parent family have different experiences of growing up; and you may have experience of being a parent, aunt or grandfather, etc.

- **Your marital status** Being married, living with a partner, divorced or widowed each bring different experiences.

- **Your gender** Boys and girls are usually brought up differently and men and women often experience different roles in the family and the workplace.

- **Your education and employment** Different people learn different things at school, experience different degrees of success in their studies, and work in jobs with different amounts of pay and status.

- **Your ethnic and cultural background** People have different experiences according to their skin colour, religious beliefs, cultural values and so on.

- **Your social class** People living in run-down areas and poor quality housing and who are on low incomes have very different experiences from people who are higher up the social ladder.

- **Your age** How old you are and the period of time you have lived through affect your views, expectations, knowledge and understanding of life.

- **Your health and ability** People with a long-term illness, a physical disability or a sensory impairment have very different experiences from people who are healthy and able-bodied.

All these different experiences combine to make us the unique individuals that we are. Because we are all unique, it is no wonder that we all prefer, wish for and need different things! The people you support are equally unique so it follows that they have their own individual preferences, wishes and needs. It is your role to be interested in and learn as much as

CASE STUDY: *Dennis and Sunil*

Dennis and Sunil are both in their late seventies and need support with maintaining their appearance, communicating and getting about. Dennis is English and Sunil comes from India. Both have worked in a London hospital all their lives – Dennis as a porter and Sunil as a doctor. Sunil is a widower with three grown up children; Dennis has never been married.

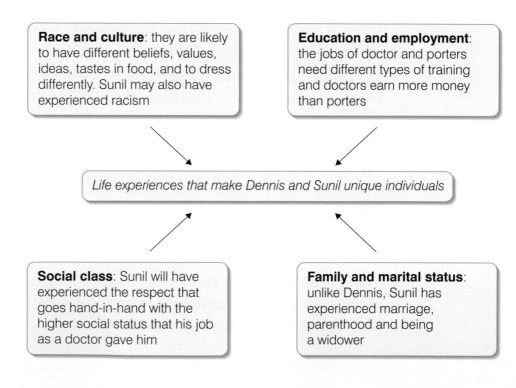

Race and culture: they are likely to have different beliefs, values, ideas, tastes in food, and to dress differently. Sunil may also have experienced racism

Education and employment: the jobs of doctor and porters need different types of training and doctors earn more money than porters

Life experiences that make Dennis and Sunil unique individuals

Social class: Sunil will have experienced the respect that goes hand-in-hand with the higher social status that his job as a doctor gave him

Family and marital status: unlike Dennis, Sunil has experienced marriage, parenthood and being a widower

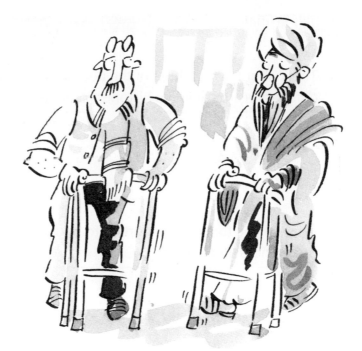

Make yourself aware of people's different needs

you can about them. When you know and understand them fully, you will be better able to care for them appropriately.

These two gentlemen are alike in that they have similar care needs, they are a similar age and they are both male. However, their very different life experiences have made them unique individuals.

Because of their different life experiences, Dennis and Sunil are likely to have different preferences, wishes and needs about the way they are supported. This doesn't mean that they should be given different standards of care. It simply means that the way they are cared for should, as far as possible, meet their needs in ways that show respect for their preferences, wishes and needs.

ACTIVITY 8

1 Think about two or three of the people you support. How do they differ as regards their life histories, preferences, wishes and needs?

2 Why do you think it is important to find out about their life histories, preferences and wishes?

1.3.3 Understand the need to make sure everything you do is based around the individual(s) you are supporting

CASE STUDY: *The Elms*

The Elms is a day care centre that aims to support people who live alone in their own homes. The care workers at The Elms have had no training in a person centred approach to care. For example, their work procedures and routines are more important to them than the people they support. They have no consideration for the preferences, wishes and needs of the people they support, and because they are inflexible in the way they work they treat everyone the same. They don't encourage the people they support to make contributions to the running of the centre; and because they clock-watch and want an easy life, they take over and do everything for the people they support.

Treating people like this is unacceptable. It makes them feel they don't matter and causes them to lose interest in themselves and their surroundings. It shows no respect for their individuality and life experiences; it denies them their independence and it doesn't promote effective work partnerships.

What do you think?

1.3.3

ACTIVITY 9

1 Think about the way you work with the people you support. Do you always make sure that your work with them is based around them and not you or the organisation you work for?

2 How can you improve the way you work to let people know that they and their care needs matter to you?

3 Why is it important to make sure that everything you do is based around the people you support?

1.3.4 Understand the need to enable the individual(s) you support to control their own lives and make informed choices about the services they receive

Think about the numerous choices that you are able to make. How would you feel if you were no longer able to make your own decisions? Frustrated? Would you feel that you are no longer in charge of your life?

Many people who use caring services find it increasingly difficult to make decisions. As a result, they become dependent on others and lose control of their lives. They feel worthless and depressed, sometimes quite devastated; and they worry about their future. Your role is to support their right to choice by encouraging them to make informed choices and regain control. Staying in control builds confidence, happiness, independence and self-esteem. It allows people to live as they choose.

CASE STUDY: Elsie

Elsie, who is 74 and lives alone, is losing her sight and her ability to understand and make decisions. Her son Tom is very worried about her and feels he has a duty to do everything for her, including bathing and dressing her, choosing what she eats, when she eats and when she goes to bed. He has also advertised for someone to clean, shop and cook for her when he is at work.

Tom is a good son – he wants to help his mother and she, no doubt, benefits from his care and support. However, he is not encouraging her to make her own choices and stay in control of her life.

You may work with people like Elsie, who are losing their ability to make choices and stay in control. In situations like this, your role is to provide them with information that they can understand and use to make informed choices, for example about what to eat, what to wear, where to go, what to watch on the television, when to get up and go to bed and how to spend their money.

It is particularly important that the people you support are able to make informed choices about their care. As you read earlier, they have a right to be cared for in ways that meet their needs and take account of their choices. Giving them an opportunity to choose the care and support they want and need helps put them in control of their care, which builds their confidence. It also acknowledges that they know more about their needs than anyone else, which builds their self-esteem. Your role is to provide the people you support with information so that they can make an informed choice about:

- the care and support services that will meet their needs
- how their care and support will be provided
- how their care can be improved or changed to meet their changing needs.

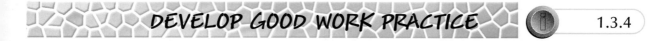

DEVELOP GOOD WORK PRACTICE
1.3.4

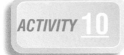

ACTIVITY 10

1 Think about two or three of the people you support who have difficulty making decisions and who are not in control of their lives. Describe the methods you currently use to help them make informed choices and to stay in control.

2 Explain how you can improve your work practice to ensure that they are able to make informed choices about the care and support they receive and remain in control.

1.3.5 Know how to use an individual's care plan when providing support

People in need of care and support are assessed to find out what care needs they have. Care needs can be:

- physical, e.g. health care, dietary, mobility and sensory needs
- intellectual, e.g. learning, memory and communication needs
- emotional, e.g. confidence, self-esteem and mental health needs
- social, e.g. needs caused by loneliness and isolation.

Care plans spell out how, where, when and by whom care needs will be met. They are agreed by the people needing support, their <u>carers</u>, e.g. family and friends, and the organisations that will be delivering the care. A <u>care package</u> is a package of services supplied by a range of organisations that provide caring services.

Care plans, which are exclusive to the people they are written for, are based on all of their needs. They also take account of people's personal preferences for how care should be given. The most important part of

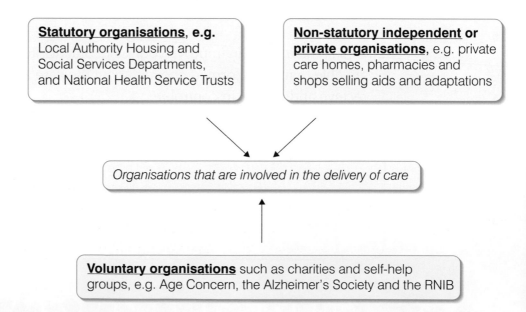

Statutory organisations, e.g. Local Authority Housing and Social Services Departments, and National Health Service Trusts

Non-statutory independent or **private organisations**, e.g. private care homes, pharmacies and shops selling aids and adaptations

Organisations that are involved in the delivery of care

Voluntary organisations such as charities and self-help groups, e.g. Age Concern, the Alzheimer's Society and the RNIB

your job is to work with people to help meet their care needs. To do this you must follow their care plans accurately and precisely. Your line manager will keep a check on how effective you are at following care plans by observing you at work and asking you questions.

You may be asked to tell your line manager how you have followed a care plan. Alternatively, you may have to make notes in care plans that describe any activities you have carried out. If you do, remember that your notes must be:

● easy to read and understand

● relevant and to the point

● factual and accurate

● checkable

● signed and dated.

In addition to following care plans, it is also your responsibility to watch out for changes in people's needs and circumstances.

Needs	How people's needs can change
Physical needs	They can find it increasingly difficult to move around, use the toilet, take their medication
Intellectual needs	They can become confused and lose interest in the world around them
Emotional needs	They can become withdrawn and depressed
Social needs	They can lose interest in maintaining relationships; friends and family may not visit as often as they used to

Changes like these are responded to by care plan reviews. You have an important role to play in the care plan review process. You may not be involved in care plan review meetings at this stage in your career but it is your responsibility to tell your line manager if you think the needs of the people you support have changed and how you and they think their care can be improved.

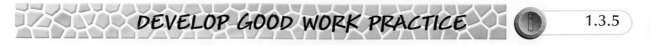

DEVELOP GOOD WORK PRACTICE
1.3.5

ACTIVITY 11

Ask your line manager to monitor your ability to use care plans when you are providing support and to sign the Witness Statement to indicate your competence.

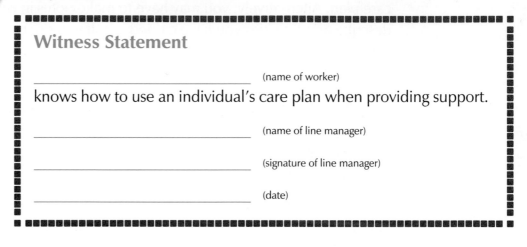

Witness Statement

_____ (name of worker)

knows how to use an individual's care plan when providing support.

_____ (name of line manager)

_____ (signature of line manager)

_____ (date)

1.4 RISK ASSESSMENT

1.4.1 Recognise that the individual(s) you support have the right to take risks

We all take risks on a daily basis, for example when we cross the road, drive a car, use alcohol – the list is endless! By taking risks we can access opportunities, such as using health and care services, being in employment and having a social life. As children, our parents and carers protected us from taking risks that could cause us harm. As adolescents, we started to become independent and learn to take and manage risks. As adults, we have a better understanding of the dangers associated with taking risks and generally only take risks we are comfortable with.

We have a right to take risks. But we also have a responsibility to protect the health and safety of ourselves and other people. It follows that behaviour that presents a risk of harm to ourselves and others is irresponsible. We have to balance our right to take risks with our health and safety responsibilities.

The people you support also have a right to take risks. Unfortunately, their ability to take risks is often restricted because other people:

- are anxious about their vulnerability to, for example, exploitation and harm
- think that if they take risks, they pose a risk to other people.

Consider the following scenarios, which show how well-meaning people treat people who need support as health and safety risks.

CASE STUDY: *Taking Risks*

A disabled woman had her request for a grab rail to help her walk from the garden gate to her front door turned down by social services because she was frail and might fall while using it.

Wheelchair users, people with mobility problems and people with sight impairments are sometimes refused admission to, for example, cinemas and theatres because they are a 'fire hazard', the argument being that it would be impossibly difficult to get them out of a building in the event of a fire.

Source: www.disabilitydebate.org/about_the_debate/discussion_papers/whose_risk_is_it_anyway.aspx

---

By labelling people who need support as a health and safety risk, either to themselves or others, we deny them opportunities that other people can access, e.g. to walk in the garden and to watch a film or a play. Denying people access to equal opportunities is a form of discrimination, which, as you know, is against the law.

Denying people who need support access to equal opportunities also restricts their ability to make choices. There may be risks attached to what they choose to do but we must never assume that they aren't able to make a sound judgement about the risks they are able and prepared to take. Denying someone the opportunity to make their own choices flies in the face of person centred care and is therefore bad care practice.

You have a responsibility to support people's rights to:

- take risks
- be protected from harm.

Eliminating risks might ensure health and safety but it takes away choice and independence. Enabling people to take risks shows respect for their preferences, wishes and needs, and helps them stay in control of their lives – but might involve a risk of harm. The risk assessment process, which you will read about in the next section, helps to identify and manage risks.

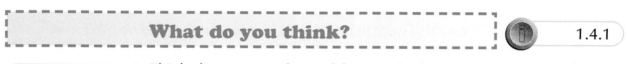

What do you think?   1.4.1

ACTIVITY 12

1 Think about two or three of the people you support. What would they like to do but are prevented from doing because of health and safety issues?

2 How do you think this affects them?

1.4.2 Understand how to use your organisation's risk assessment procedures to assess whether the behaviour/activities of the individual(s) you support present a risk of harm to themselves or others

Risk assessment enables people to make choices and access opportunities safely. The risk assessment process involves:

Step 1: Identifying behaviours and activities that are <u>hazardous</u> and could put people's health and safety at risk

Step 2: Deciding who might be harmed and how

Step 3: Taking steps to minimise risks, for example by helping people choose alternative behaviours and activities that present less of a risk

Step 4: Recording hazards, risks and precautions in a risk assessment procedure document for the benefit of everyone involved

Step 5: Regularly reviewing hazards, risks and precautions and updating procedures as appropriate.

You have a responsibility to follow risk assessment procedures and to continually check whether people's behaviour and activities present a risk of harm to themselves or others. Watch out for evidence of:

- **deliberate self harm** – for example because they have mental ill health, suicidal thoughts or abuse alcohol or drugs

- **accidental self harm** – for example because they live in an unsafe, insecure environment, they neglect themselves, they are becoming increasingly frail, they are losing their social and intellectual skills, they fail to use their mobility equipment or <u>aids and adaptations</u>, they are anxious or they abuse alcohol or drugs

- **people who are at risk of harm from others** – for example from abusive or challenging behaviour or because their frailty and failing intellectual and inappropriate social skills make them vulnerable

- **people who are at risk of harm to others** – for example because they are aggressive or have a history of violence, they have failing social and intellectual skills, they abuse alcohol or drugs, they have mental ill health or they have expressed a desire to harm others.

DEVELOP GOOD WORK PRACTICE

1.4.2

ACTIVITY 13

Ask your line manager to monitor your ability to use risk assessment procedures to assess whether the behaviour/activities of the individual(s) you support present a risk of harm to themselves or others and to sign the Witness Statement to indicate your competence.

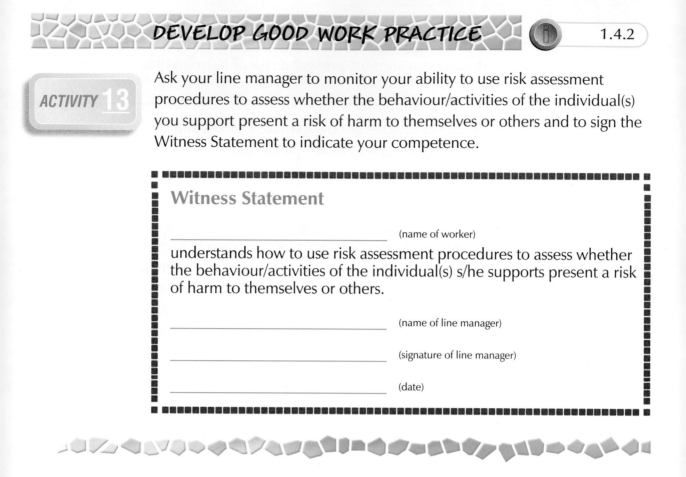

Witness Statement

_____ (name of worker)

understands how to use risk assessment procedures to assess whether the behaviour/activities of the individual(s) s/he supports present a risk of harm to themselves or others.

_____ (name of line manager)

_____ (signature of line manager)

_____ (date)

1.4.3   Know how to inform relevant people about any risks identified

Evidence of any health and safety risks that concern you must be reported without delay. Alerting colleagues to new or changing hazards ensures that risks can be minimised and precautions reviewed, which in turn upholds people's right to behave in the way they choose.

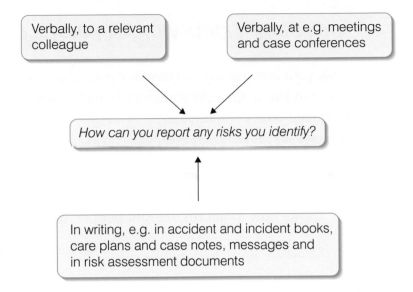

How and to whom should you report the risks you identify? Each organisation has its own procedure for reporting risks. Make sure you are familiar with your organisation's procedures and that you follow them.

As a rule of thumb, report your concerns as soon as possible, before you forget them; and if you put them in writing, make sure that what you write is:

- easy to read and understand
- relevant and to the point
- factual and accurate
- checkable
- signed and dated.

DEVELOP GOOD WORK PRACTICE

1.4.3

ACTIVITY 14

Ask your line manager to monitor your ability to inform the relevant people about any risks you identify and to sign the Witness Statement to indicate your competence.

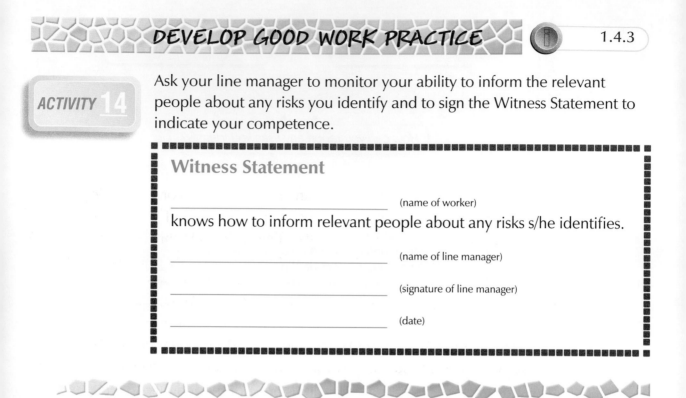

Witness Statement

_____ (name of worker)

knows how to inform relevant people about any risks s/he identifies.

_____ (name of line manager)

_____ (signature of line manager)

_____ (date)

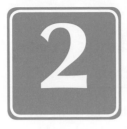

2 Understand the organisation and the role of the worker

For care workers to deliver care and support professionally and in the way that is required of them, they need to understand their <u>job role</u> and to have a knowledge and understanding of their organisation's aims and values. They need to know the importance of working with other people, including colleagues and people who are important to service users, such as carers and <u>advocates</u>. They need to understand the importance of following policies and procedures, being reliable and dependable, and the responsibilities and limits of their relationships with the people they support. This chapter aims to develop your knowledge and understanding of these issues so that you can develop work practices that support the care, safety and well being of the individuals you work with.

Successful completion of the activities in this chapter will enable you to demonstrate your understanding of the Common Induction Standard *Understand the organisation and the role of the worker*. It will also give you an opportunity to develop evidence for key skills unit Communication at level I.

What is covered in this chapter?

This chapter contributes to the knowledge and understanding you need for the following NVQ Care units at level 2:

HSC 21 : Communicate with, and complete records for individuals

HSC 22 : Support the health and safety of yourself and individuals

HSC 23 : Develop your knowledge and practice

HSC 24 : Ensure your own actions support the care, protection and well being of individuals

2.1 YOUR ROLE AS A WORKER

2.1.1 Understand your responsibilities as outlined in the GSCC Code of Practice for Social Care Workers

The General Social Care Council (GSCC) works to raise standards in social care. It regulates or controls the social care workforce in England and is responsible for:

- the Codes of Practice for social care workers (see below) and employers. These set out the standards of practice and conduct that everyone working in social care should meet.

- the Social Care Register. At the time of writing (September 2006) the register is only open to qualified social workers but everyone who works in social care in England will be required to join in the future. People who register must abide by the Code of Practice for Social Care Workers; if they breach the Code of Practice they can be removed from the register and lose their job.

- social work education and training.

The Care Council for Wales (CCW), the Scottish Social Services Council (SSSC) and the Social Services Inspectorate (SSI) for Northern Ireland perform the same functions as the GSCC in Wales, Scotland and Northern Ireland respectively.

It is very important that you understand your responsibilities as set out in the Code of Practice for Social Care Workers. The Code guides you in your work and lets you know what standards of conduct your employer, colleagues, the people you support, carers and the public expect of you. You should also use the Code of Practice to examine the way you work and to look for areas in which you can improve.

The following table sums up your responsibilities as set out in the GSCC Code of Practice. Some you will be already familiar with; others will be explained to you in following sections.

1 You must protect the rights and promote the interests of the people you support and carers	1.1 Treat each person as an individual 1.2 Respect and, where appropriate, promote their individual views and wishes 1.3 Support their rights to control their lives and make informed choices about the services they receive 1.4 Respect and maintain their dignity and privacy 1.5 Promote equal opportunities 1.6 Respect diversity and different cultures and values
2 You must strive to establish and maintain the trust and confidence of the people you support and carers	2.1 Be honest and trustworthy 2.2 Communicate in an appropriate, open, accurate and straightforward way 2.3 Respect confidential information and clearly explain your organisation's policies about confidentiality 2.4 Be reliable and dependable 2.5 Honour work commitments, agreements and arrangements and, when it is not possible to do so, explain why 2.6 Declare issues that might create conflict of interest and make sure that they do not influence your judgement or practice 2.7 Adhere to policies and procedures about accepting gifts and money
3 You must promote the independence of people you support while protecting them as far as possible from danger or harm	3.1 Promote their independence and assist them to understand and exercise their rights 3.2 Use established processes and procedures to challenge and report dangerous, abusive, discriminatory or exploitative behaviour and practice 3.3 Follow practice and procedures designed to keep you and other people safe from violent and abusive behaviour at work 3.4 Bring to the attention of your employer or the appropriate authority any resource or operational difficulties that might get in the way of the delivery of safe care 3.5 Inform your employer or an appropriate authority where the practice of colleagues may be unsafe or adversely affecting standards of care 3.6 Comply with employers' health and safety policies, including those relating to substance abuse 3.7 Help them to make complaints, take complaints seriously and respond to them or pass them to the appropriate person 3.8 Recognise and use responsibly the power that comes from your work with them
4 You must respect the rights of the people you support while seeking to ensure that their behaviour does not harm themselves or other people	4.1 Recognise that they have the right to take risks and help them to identify and manage potential and actual risks to themselves and others 4.2 Follow risk assessment policies and procedures to assess whether their behaviour presents a risk of harm to themselves or others 4.3 Take necessary steps to minimise the risks of service users from doing actual or potential harm to themselves or other people 4.4 Ensure that relevant colleagues and agencies are informed about the outcomes and implications of risk assessments

5 You must uphold public trust and confidence in social care services	5.1 You must not abuse, neglect or harm the people you support, carers or colleagues
	5.2 You must not exploit the people you support, carers or colleagues in any way
	5.3 You must not abuse the trust of the people you support and carers or the access you have to personal information about them or to their property, home or workplace
	5.4 You must not form inappropriate relationships with the people you support
	5.5 You must not discriminate unlawfully or unjustifiably against the people you support, carers or their colleagues
	5.6 You must not condone any unlawful or unjustifiable discrimination by the people you support, carers or colleagues
	5.7 You must not put yourself or others at unnecessary risk
	5.8 You must not behave in a way, in work or outside work, which would call into question your suitability to work in social services
6 You must be accountable for the quality of your work and take responsibility for maintaining and improving your knowledge and skills	6.1 Meet relevant standards of practice and work in a lawful, safe and effective way
	6.2 Maintain clear and accurate records as required by procedures established for your work
	6.3 Inform your employer or the appropriate authority about any personal difficulties that might affect your ability to do your job competently and safely
	6.4 Seek assistance from your employer or the appropriate authority if you do not feel able or adequately prepared to carry out any aspect of your work, or you are not sure about how to proceed in a work matter
	6.5 Work openly and co-operatively with colleagues and treat them with respect
	6.6 Recognise that you remain responsible for the work that you delegate to other workers
	6.7 Recognise and respect the roles and expertise of workers from other organisations and work in partnership with them
	6.8 Undertake relevant training to maintain and improve your knowledge and skills, and contribute to the learning and development of others

Source: www.gscc.org.uk/Good+practice+and+conduct/Get+copies+of+our+codes/

CHECK YOUR UNDERSTANDING

2.1.1

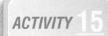

Produce an illustrated poster to display in your staff room that describes the GSCC Code of Practice for Social Care Workers.

2.1.2 Understand your job role in relation to the aims and values of the organisation

All organisations have aims or goals and everyone employed in an organisation is expected to work together to achieve those aims. Organisations also have values or beliefs about how their aims are to be achieved.

For care workers to carry out their job roles effectively they need to know and understand their organisation's aims and values. Most organisations that provide caring services sum up their aims in Mission Statements and/or Charters of Care. Mission Statements and Charters of Care also tell us what an organisation's beliefs or values are by describing how they provide the service. An example of a mission statement that describes an organisation's aim and values is:

> *Our aim is to provide the people we support with care and support in ways that encourage them to be independent and make choices and that respect their individuality, privacy and dignity.*

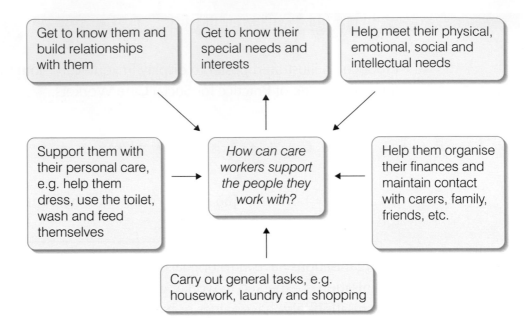

Your job may involve these activities and many more besides! Your responsibility in making sure that your organisation achieves its aims and values is to:

- use the principles of care in your work (see Chapter 1)
- follow the GSCC Code of Practice (see the previous section)
- use the GSCC Code of Practice to examine the way you work and to look for areas in which you can improve. You will learn how to improve your knowledge and skills in Chapter 6
- follow your organisation's work procedures, which as you know are based on laws and the GSCC Code of Practice
- work in such a way that risks to health and safety are minimised. You will learn how to maintain health and safety in Chapter 3
- use support and supervision effectively. You will learn about support and supervision in Chapter 6.

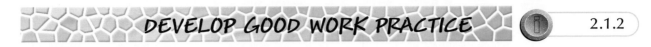

DEVELOP GOOD WORK PRACTICE

2.1.2

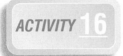

Describe your organisation's aims and values. Your line manager will be able to tell you what they are or there may be a Mission Statement or Charter of Care that you can read.

Now use the table below to describe 3 of your work activities and how you should carry each out to help your organisation meet its aims and values.

Work activities	How the way I work helps my organisation meet its aims and values

2.1.3 Understand the roles of other workers and the importance of working in partnership with them

When you applied for your job, you were probably asked how you get on with other people. This is because care workers need to be interested in other people, enjoy their company and be able to work with them.

Care workers work in partnership or in teams with the people they support, their family, friends and carers, and their colleagues. They also work with social care teams such as porters, social workers and occupational therapists. Other teams that they are likely to have contact with include:

- caretaking teams, e.g. gardeners, odd job people, security staff
- domestic teams, e.g. cleaners, kitchen and laundry staff
- health care teams, e.g. health care assistants, nurses, doctors, physiotherapists
- management and administration teams.

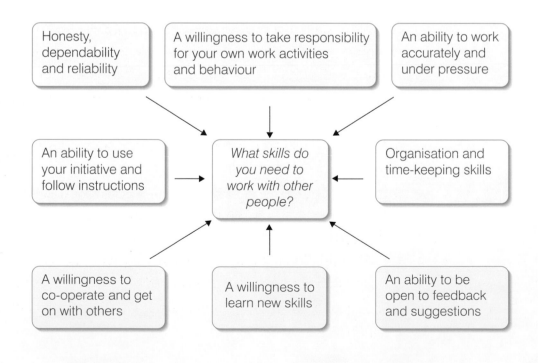

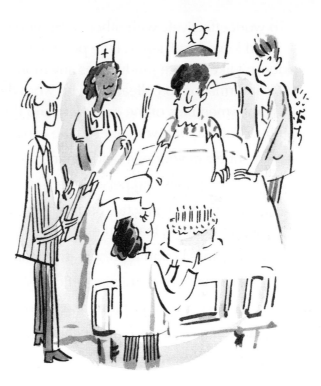

Each person has a valuable role to play in providing care

Each team is equally important and one team cannot function without the support of others. As a care worker you play a very important role in working with your own and other teams of workers, for example:

- your own team cannot meet people's care needs if you don't carry out your job role as required
- the kitchen team cannot do its job without your instructions about individual dietary needs
- the health care team cannot meet health needs if you don't encourage the people you support to take their medication and let you know how they feel
- the occupational therapy team can only be effective if you make them aware of any day-to-day problems that individuals experience
- the security team cannot maintain a secure environment unless you report your concerns.

To work effectively with other teams you need to understand their varied job roles. There is little point telling admin staff that Mrs Jackson doesn't like cheese sandwiches any more; it is only necessary to give this information to colleagues who work directly with Mrs Jackson, such as other members of the care team and the kitchen staff. Sources of information about work roles in the caring services include:

- members of your own and other teams
- job descriptions and person specifications
- official codes of practice and standards produced by, e.g. the Department of Health, the GSCC and Skills for Care
- your Trades Union representative/learning representative
- your organisation's training officer/NVQ assessor
- specialist care publications, e.g. journals, magazines, books
- professional organisations such as the Care Homes Association
- the Commission for Social Care Inspection.

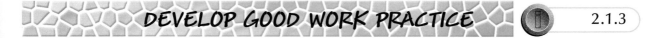

DEVELOP GOOD WORK PRACTICE
2.1.3

ACTIVITY 17

1 Talk to four or five people that you work with on a day-to-day basis about their work and write a job description for each person.

2   Why is it important that you work in partnership with each of these workers?

2.1.4 Understand the value and importance of working in partnership with unpaid carers/advocates/significant others

People who care for others on an informal, unpaid basis are known as carers. They include family, friends, and people who volunteer for charitable organisations like Age Concern and the Alzheimer's Society. Advocates are individuals who speak up on behalf of people who need support because, for one reason or another, they cannot speak up for themselves. They also often work on a voluntary basis for charitable organisations. 'Significant others' is a term used to describe individuals who are important to people who need support. They are usually family and friends but also include people in their community and social circle such as fellow worshippers, bowls partners, drinking pals, the milkman and the window cleaner.

People who need support, their carers, advocates and significant others are very important to each other. They need to feel loved and valued by each other; they need to be able to give love and show how much they appreciate each other; and they need the security of continuing to be in a relationship with each other. For these reasons it is extremely important to include carers, advocates and significant others in the day-to-day lives of the people you support.

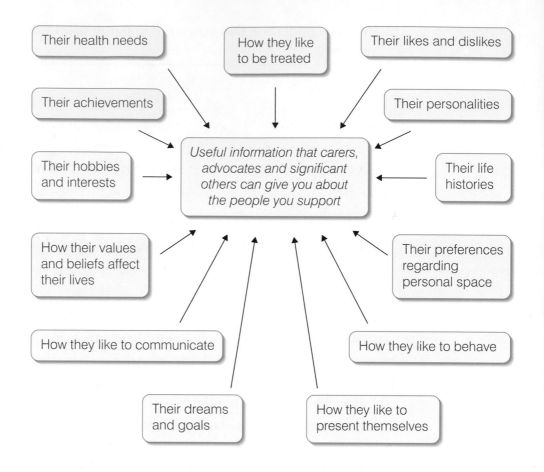

In addition to meeting the needs for love, companionship and security, carers, advocates and significant others can help you in your work by giving you information that the people you support might not think to tell you.

Having information like this helps you to:

- get to know and understand the people you support as individuals
- care for them in ways that meet their needs and take account of their preferences and choices
- promote their rights
- demonstrate respect for their values and cultural background
- support their equal opportunities
- promote their dignity and privacy.

In other words, it enables you to use the principles of care in your work.

Involving carers, advocates and significant others in the care team and developing relationships with them also helps protect the people you support from neglect or abuse. Open, trusting relationships in which care workers, carers, advocates and significant others can voice their concerns help identify and prevent behaviour which may become abusive or neglectful. You will read about abuse and neglect in Chapter 5.

How can you involve carers, advocates and significant others in the day-to-day lives of the people you support? You could:

- invite them to meetings, for example care planning meetings
- ask them for ideas for parties and outings and when you are organising hobby and interest groups
- ask them about activities, for example to celebrate religious festivals
- suggest they might like to set up support groups
- invite them to set up mixed faith groups for discussion and worship
- organise visits to schools attended by young relatives
- organise visits to concerts, places of worship, shops, pubs, etc. in the community.

You could also talk with your line manager about making sure that your organisation has an 'open-door' policy, so that carers, advocates and significant others are able to talk to the care team at any time.

CHECK YOUR UNDERSTANDING

2.1.4

ACTIVITY 18

Use the following table to note down three examples of how your organisation involves carers, advocates and significant others in the day-to-day lives of the people you support, and to describe how their involvement benefits everyone concerned.

How carers, advocates and significant others are involved in the day-to-day lives of the people I support	How their involvement benefits everyone concerned
1	
2	
3	

2.2 POLICIES AND PROCEDURES

2.2.1 Understand why it is important for you to follow policies and procedures

A *policy* is an official document that gives information about *what* must be done within a particular organisation such as a social care service provider. It sets out the organisation's responsibilities by describing the standards that workers have to use in their work. Organisations have a number of policies, each one ensuring that one or more different laws are obeyed. For example:

- Health and Safety Policies contain information about the standards of safe and healthy working that workers must follow in their activities. They also spell out workers' responsibilities in making sure that health and safety laws and regulations are obeyed.

A *procedure* is an official document that explains to workers *how* they must do their work, i.e. it translates or interprets policies into working methods. Procedures also explain how workers must use their organisation's beliefs or values in their work. For example:

- A Health and Safety Policy will include information about the standards of working to be followed when dealing with hazardous substances such as cleaning materials and bodily waste. The appropriate Health and Safety Procedure will describe exactly how to work with, e.g. bleach, blood and urine.

It is most important that you follow your organisation's policies and procedures, for the following reasons:

- to encourage and maintain good, safe working practices that promote rights and apply the principles of care
- to build and maintain your organisation's reputation as a highly regarded service provider. You and the people you support benefit from being associated with an organisation that has a good reputation
- to obey the law. If an organisation is found to be disobeying the law, it can be closed down. Similarly, it is your responsibility to know what the law says as you can be held legally responsible if your actions,

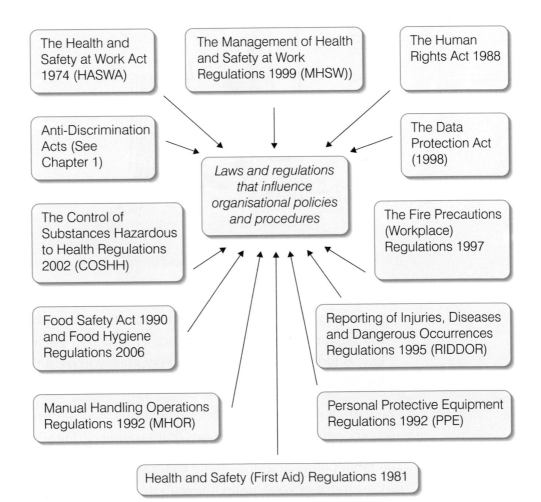

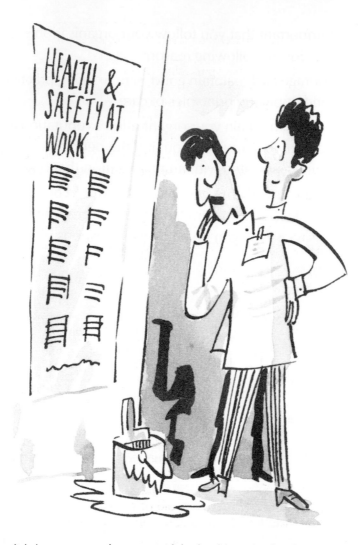

It is important to be aware of the health and safety laws and regulations

omissions (what you don't do but should), errors or blunders result in things going wrong at work. Ignorance is no excuse in the eyes of the law. A judge wouldn't let you off because you didn't know you had to tax and insure your car.

There are a number of laws and regulations that determine the policies and procedures for organisations that provide caring services.

The table below describes some examples of organisational policies and procedures that you should know about.

Policies and procedures	What the policies and procedures cover
Health and safety	Everyone's responsibilities in helping to keep the workplace free from health and safety risks Everyone's rights to information and training about health and safety issues
Responding to abuse	What to do when there is a risk of abuse, what to do after an abusive incident and how to report and record abuse Everyone's rights to support and to training on how to recognise and deal with abuse
Confidentiality and disclosure of information	What information must be kept confidential, where it should be stored, who it may be disclosed to and why
Control of exposure to hazardous waste	Whether waste is hazardous or not, the health and safety risks of working with hazardous waste, how to protect against risks, how to dispose of waste safely and what to do if there is an accident involving hazardous waste
Fire safety	What to do to prevent fire and the emergency action to take if there is a fire
Hygiene and food safety	Safe and hygienic food storage, preparation, cooking and serving in order to protect against food poisoning
Moving and handling	The need to assess (check) moving and handling risks They also describe safe ways to move and handle loads, including the people you support
Dealing with accidents and emergencies	The need to have named, qualified first-aiders in the workplace, how to send for the emergency health services and how to record accidents and injuries What should be in the first aid box and who is responsible for maintaining the first aid box. Also about ensuring training in first aid
Infection control	Precautions to be taken when working with people who have infectious diseases. Also about whether infections need to be reported and who to
Record keeping and access to files	Everyone's responsibilities to report, record and file information as requested by the line manager or manager
Complaints and comments	How to make a complaint and how complaints must be dealt with

2.2.1

ACTIVITY 19

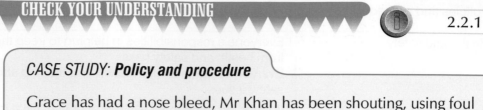

CASE STUDY: *Policy and procedure*

Grace has had a nose bleed, Mr Khan has been shouting, using foul language and upsetting the residents, and one of your colleagues has tripped and fallen.

1 What documents would tell you how to deal with these situations?

2 What documents would contain information about the standards of work you are expected to follow in dealing with these situations?

3 Why is it important that you follow policies and procedures when dealing with these situations?

2.2.2 Know how to access a full list and up-to-date copy of all organisational policies and procedures

Find out where your organisation's policies and procedures are kept. Most workplaces store them in files or folders in a central office where they can be easily accessed. Study the ones that affect you and make sure you use them in your work. If there is anything you don't understand, ask a colleague or your line manager.

Organisational policies and procedures are regularly updated because, for example:

- laws and regulations are amended from time to time
- research shows that care practice needs to change, e.g. the NHS Modernisation Agency identified that staff need to change the way they work with people in order to maintain their privacy and dignity
- advances in technology lead to the development of new methods of, for example, giving medication, helping someone to move, and new equipment for measuring temperature, sugar levels and blood pressure, and so on.

It is your responsibility to keep up with changes in your organisation's policies and procedures and to adapt your methods of working as required. Don't forget, if you make mistakes because you don't follow correct procedures, you can be held legally responsible!

CHECK YOUR UNDERSTANDING   2.2.2

ACTIVITY 20

Produce an information leaflet for someone like yourself who is new to care work that describes:

- where your workplace policies and procedures are stored
- who is responsible for updating them
- the reasons why they may have to be updated.

2.3 WORKER RELATIONSHIPS

2.3.1 Understand the responsibilities and limits of your relationship with the individual(s) you support

Think about the people you know and with whom you have relationships. If you were to make a list of the relationships you have, you might include:

- family relationships
- friendships
- sexual relationships
- working relationships.

Good relationships are very important. Family, friends, sexual partners and work colleagues, in one way or another, offer each other companionship, advice, support, a sense of belonging and the opportunity to share experiences, such as a day out shopping or an evening at the pub. As a result of having good relationships we feel valued and cared for.

Because care workers work *with* the people they support, the relationship between them is a working relationship. Friendships might form; and there are instances where care workers and the people they work with have fallen in love and settled down together. But, as a rule of thumb, because you are employed to work with the people you support, the relationship that develops between you must be different from a friendship, family or sexual relationship.

CASE STUDY: *Lena and Bessie*

Lena and Bessie have been friends for years. They have been there for each other through thick and thin. Until recently, that is, when Bessie heard on the grapevine that Lena had been talking about her behind her back, criticising her and spreading rumours about her that are hurtful and untrue.

Friendships can go sour. Do you think that this sort of behaviour would be acceptable if Lena was Bessie's care worker? No, it wouldn't. Lena's behaviour doesn't show any value for the relationship she had shared with Bessie or any respect for what had been confidential between them.

Think back to the case study earlier about Elsie, whose son Tom feels he has a duty to do everything for her, including bathing and dressing her, choosing what and when she will eat, when she will go to bed and who will clean, shop and cook for her when he is at work.

Do you think care workers should behave like this with the people they support? No, because this sort of behaviour does not promote privacy, dignity, partnership and equal opportunities, and it does not encourage people to make their own choices, stay in control or take risks.

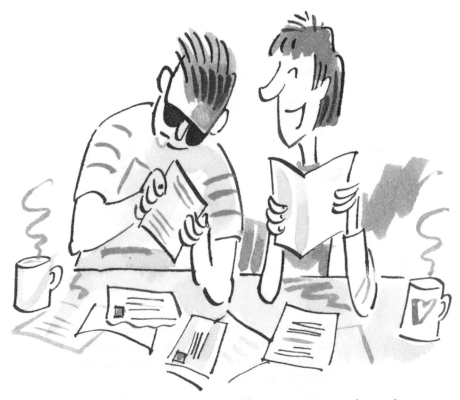

A professional relationship must be maintained between a care worker and a service user

CASE STUDY: *Carla*

Carla is very supportive of her neighbour Jack, who has multiple sclerosis. Recently Jack asked her if she would help him have a bath. Because they have been such good friends for a long time, Carla agreed to help and one thing led to another ...

This is the stuff that movies are made of! But do you think that having a sexual relationship with someone you support is appropriate behaviour for a paid care worker? No, it isn't. Sexual relationships bring people very close emotionally and emotions can prevent people giving professional, person centred care.

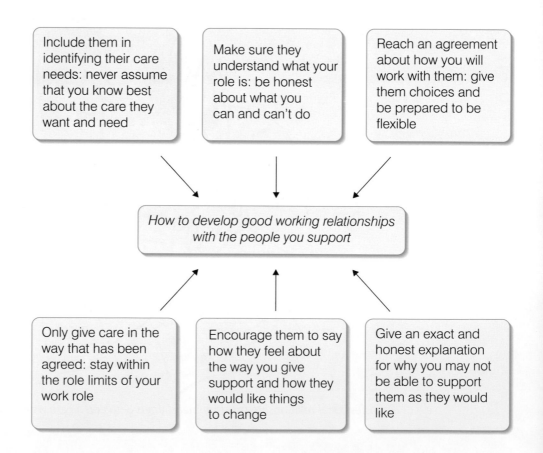

Include them in identifying their care needs: never assume that you know best about the care they want and need

Make sure they understand what your role is: be honest about what you can and can't do

Reach an agreement about how you will work with them: give them choices and be prepared to be flexible

How to develop good working relationships with the people you support

Only give care in the way that has been agreed: stay within the role limits of your work role

Encourage them to say how they feel about the way you give support and how they would like things to change

Give an exact and honest explanation for why you may not be able to support them as they would like

Caring relationships between friends, family members and sexual partners can lack one or other of the principles of care. As a care worker your responsibility is to develop working relationships with the people you support, which avoid the drawbacks of personal relationships and in which you can:

- apply the principles of care
- follow policies and procedures
- maintain standards as outlined in the GSCC Code of Practice.

CHECK YOUR UNDERSTANDING

2.3.1

ACTIVITY 21

CASE STUDY: *Abdul*

Abdul has recently moved into The Beeches Residential Home. Bob, a care worker, has told Abdul not to worry, he won't have to say a word because Bob knows exactly what his residents are thinking and what they need. And if Abdul wants anything doing at any time of the day or night, he'll be there to do it for him.

Explain how Bob's behaviour is unacceptable in terms of his relationship with Abdul.

2.3.2 Understand the need to be reliable and dependable

Being reliable and dependable means always doing what you say you are going to do and always doing what you are expected to do. It means being responsible, committed and loyal. If you are reliable and dependable, people will trust you and have confidence in you.

As a care worker, you must strive to establish and maintain the trust and confidence of the people you support and their carers (see the GSCC Codes of Practice). You must also strive to establish and maintain the trust and confidence of your colleagues.

CASE STUDY: *Mrs Crabtree, Elliot and Jacqui*

Mrs Crabtree needs to use the toilet. Two or three care workers promised to take her, but none of them has kept their promise.

Elliot's daughter has rung in to say she won't be able to visit him as arranged. The care worker who took the call fails to let Elliot know.

Jacqui is regularly late for work, takes time off for unacceptable reasons, doesn't work skilfully and doesn't pull her weight in a team.

Can you see how the care workers in these case studies are not reliable and dependable? And can you understand that their behaviour threatens the trust and confidence of the people they support, their carers and their colleagues?

Areas of responsibility in which it is particularly important that care workers are reliable and dependable include:

- in their work with the people they support and their carers, their colleagues and people from other organisations
- when following policies and procedures
- when using the GSCC Code of Practice and the principles of care
- when promoting and maintaining health and safety and responding to concerns about danger, harm and abuse.

ACTIVITY 22

Make notes on the following:

1 Think about four or five occasions when your friends, family or colleagues haven't been reliable and dependable. How did their behaviour make you feel?

2 Now think about four or five occasions when you haven't been particularly reliable and dependable. How do you think your behaviour affected the people concerned?

3 Why is it important to be reliable and dependable at work?

4 List five ways in which you can improve the way you work so that you
   become more reliable and dependable.

3 Maintain safety at work

It is important that care workers have a knowledge and understanding of the health and safety laws and regulations that affect how they carry out their work. It is equally important that they follow these laws and regulations. This chapter tells you about the laws and regulations that apply to working in care and how you should put them into practice. It builds on what you have learnt about the principles of care, your workplace policies and procedures and your role as a worker.

Successful completion of the activities in this chapter will allow you to demonstrate your understanding of the Common Induction Standard *Maintain safety at work*. It will also give you an opportunity to produce evidence for the key skills unit Communication at level I.

What is covered in this chapter?

This chapter contributes to the knowledge and understanding you need for the following NVQ Care units at level 2:
HSC 21 : Communicate with, and complete records for individuals
HSC 22 : Support the health and safety of yourself and individuals
HSC 23 : Develop your knowledge and practice
HSC 24 : Ensure your own actions support the care, protection and well being of individuals

3.1 HEALTH AND SAFETY

3.1.1 Be aware of key legislation relating to health and safety in your work setting(s) and understand the responsibilities of yourself, your employer and the individuals you support.

The *Health and Safety at Work Act 1974 (HASWA)* is the basis of British health and safety law. It requires employers to use common sense when identifying risks and to take sensible measures to tackle them. Workers' responsibilities under the Health and Safety at Work Act are:

- to take care of everyone who may be affected by their work, by
  - only doing work they have been trained to do
  - using and storing equipment and materials properly
  - not fooling around or taking chances or short cuts
- to report health and safety <u>hazards</u> to their line manager without delay, including
  - faulty equipment and safety signs that have been tampered with
  - blocked exits and escape routes (stairwells, fire doors)
  - infectious diseases, injuries and accidents
- to help their employer carry out their health and safety responsibilities by
  - following workplace health and safety procedures
  - not tampering with anything provided for their health and safety
  - knowing what to do in an emergency, such as a fire
  - using protective clothing and equipment correctly.

The *Management of Health and Safety at Work Regulations 1999* require employers to carry out <u>risk assessments</u>, write health and safety procedures and provide everyone with health and safety information and training in, for example, fire safety, infection control, food safety, manual handling, the use of equipment and working with hazardous materials.

The *Workplace (Health, Safety and Welfare) Regulations 1992* require employers to look after people's health, safety and welfare by providing ventilation, heating, lighting, workstations, seating and welfare facilities.

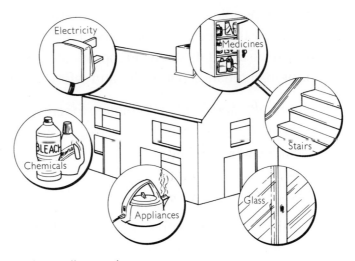

Potential hazards are all around us

The *Personal Protective Equipment at Work Regulations 1992 (PPE)* require employers to provide workers with appropriate protective equipment and clothing, such as aprons, gloves and masks. Workers have a responsibility to follow procedures regarding what to wear and to use the protective clothing and equipment they are given to, for example, prevent cross-infection.

The *Provision and Use of Work Equipment Regulations 1998 (PUWER)* require employers to make sure that equipment and machinery they provide for workers, such as electrical equipment and electronically operated devices, are safe. Workers' responsibility is to follow procedures regarding the use and maintenance of equipment and to report any concerns they have about its safety. Inappropriate use of equipment and poor maintenance put health and safety at risk.

The *Manual Handling Operations Regulations 1992 (MHOR)* require employers to write procedures for the safe moving of objects by hand or bodily force. Workers have a responsibility to follow these procedures when moving any type of load, including the people they support, to protect everyone concerned against accidents and injuries.

The *Lifting Operations and Lifting Equipment Regulations (LOLER) 1999* require employers to make sure that equipment used for moving objects, such as hoists, is safe and that everyone is trained in its use. Workers and the people they support have a responsibility to follow procedures regarding the safe use of lifting equipment and to report any concerns they have about its safety. Inappropriate use of lifting equipment and its poor maintenance put health and safety at risk.

The *Health and Safety Information for Employees Regulations 1989* require employers to display a poster telling everyone what they need to know about health and safety.

The *Reporting of Injuries, Diseases and Dangerous Occurrences Regulations 1995 (RIDDOR)* require employers to record and report certain workplace injuries, diseases and dangerous events to the relevant authorities. An organisation's procedures outline workers' responsibilities for recording and reporting injuries, diseases and dangerous events, which is necessary to help prevent them happening again.

The *Control of Substances Hazardous to Health Regulations 2002 (COSHH)* require employers to assess the risks from hazardous substances and to write safe working procedures, which are usually stored in a COSHH file. Workers' responsibility is to read the file, get to know the procedures and follow them to the letter.

The *Food Safety Act 1990* and the *Food Hygiene Regulations 2006* state that everyone who handles food has a responsibility to maintain a high standard of personal hygiene when handling food and a high standard of hygiene in areas where food is stored, prepared and cooked.

The *Health and Safety (First Aid) Regulations 1981* require employers to cover needs for first aid, for example to train staff in first aid procedures, appoint a first-aider and ensure there is someone responsible for maintaining the first aid box. Workers' responsibility is to attend first aid training, to update their first aid skills as required, to know how to send for the emergency health services and to follow procedures for reporting and recording accidents and injuries.

The *Electricity at Work Regulations 1989* and the *Gas Safety (Installation and Use) Regulations 1994* require everyone who works with gas and electrical appliances to make sure they are safe to use and are maintained in a safe condition.

CHECK YOUR UNDERSTANDING

3.1.1

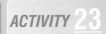

Make a list of the laws and regulations that affect health and safety where you work and list the responsibilities for health and safety that:

1 you have

2 your employer has

3 the people you support have

3.1.2 Understand your organisation's policies and procedures in relation to health and safety in your work setting(s) and the individual(s) you support

You read earlier that an organisation's policies are based on laws and regulations. You also read that procedures interpret policies into working methods. The previous section emphasised that workers have a responsibility to follow health and safety procedures. If they don't follow procedures and things go wrong, they can be held legally responsible.

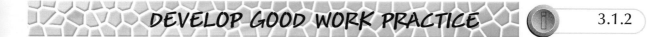

DEVELOP GOOD WORK PRACTICE   3.1.2

ACTIVITY 24

Find out about the health and safety policies and procedures that affect the way you do your job. Produce a poster for your staff room that shows you understand these policies and procedures in relation to:

- your <u>work setting</u>
- the people you support.

3.1.3 Know how to apply your organisation's policies and procedures in relation to health and safety in your work setting(s) and the individual(s) you support

This section describes some of the working methods that will help you maintain health and safety at work.

Gas leaks, electrical emergencies and water leaks

Because gas is flammable, leaks can cause fires and explosions. They can also cause breathing problems, unconsciousness and <u>asphyxiation</u>. Your organisation will have a procedure for dealing with gas leaks but as a general rule:

- turn the gas off at the mains supply (usually near the gas meter)
- turn off fires and cookers and do not light matches or cigarette lighters
- open windows and doors to let the gas escape
- telephone the emergency number of the gas company from an outside telephone (in case using the workplace telephone causes an explosion)
- if you have been trained in first aid, help people who develop breathing difficulties. If there is a health emergency, dial 999 or get help from a GP
- tell your line manager what you have done.

Power surges, exposed wires, frayed cables, faulty switches and electrical appliances are also fire risks. Electricity can cause shock, burns and asphyxiation. Again, your workplace will have a procedure for responding to electrical emergencies but as a general rule:

- turn the electricity supply off at the mains (usually near the fuse box)
- never touch a person or object that is connected to the electrical supply
- if you have been trained in first aid, help people who develop breathing difficulties or who have had an electric shock. If there is a health emergency, dial 999 or get help from a GP
- tell your line manager what you have done.

Water leaks can rot floorboards and floor coverings, making them hazardous. When water comes into contact with electricity there is a risk of fire and electrical injuries. Your workplace will have a procedure to follow in the event of a water leak, but as a general rule:

- put a bucket, bowl or towel under the leak
- turn the water supply off at the stopcock (usually near a sink)
- if water is leaking from the main water tank, leave bath taps turned on to empty the tank
- call the emergency number of the water company
- mop up as best you can.
- tell your line manager what you have done.

Working with hazardous substances

The table below describes some of the hazardous substances you might come into contact with and their effects on health.

Harzardous substances	Examples	Health effects
Cleaning materials	Bleach, disinfectant	Skin problems, e.g. burns, dermatitis; breathing problems, e.g. asthma
Body fluids and waste	Blood, vomit, mucus, urine, faeces	Infections
Clinical waste	Used dressings	Infections
Sharps	Needles, syringes	Wounds and infections
Soiled linen	Sheets, clothing	Infections

Your organisation's COSHH procedures tell you:

- what protective clothing you must wear when you work with hazardous substances, e.g. gloves and aprons
- how to store hazardous substances, e.g. in correctly labelled containers with safety lids
- how to dispose of hazardous substances:
  - body fluids and waste must be flushed down the sluice drain
  - clinical waste must be put in a labelled yellow bag and sent for incineration
  - sharps must be put in a yellow sharps box and sent for incineration
  - soiled linen must be put in red bags and sent to the laundry
  - unused medication should be returned to the pharmacist.

Hygiene

Food that is not handled safely can become contaminated (spoiled). If we eat food that has been contaminated by bacteria, we risk getting food poisoning. The symptoms of food poisoning are <u>nausea</u>, stomach pains, diarrhoea and vomiting. The people you support are most at risk of getting food poisoning, therefore you have a responsibility to know what causes it and how to prevent it happening.

The table below describes some of the bacteria that cause food poisoning.

Name of bacteria	Where the bacteria are found
Staphylococcus aureus (S.aureus)	On our skin, in our nose, throat, mouth, ears, hair, nails, and in wounds such as cuts and boils. S. aureus is relatively harmless until it is transferred to food, when it produces poisons (toxins)
Escherichia coli (E. coli)	Our intestines and our faeces. E.coli is also harmless until it is transferred to food
Salmonella and Clostridium perfringens	Raw meat, poultry, eggs, shell fish and sometimes in human faeces

As well as growing in raw food and being carried by humans, food poisoning bacteria are found in:

- pets and pests, e.g. dogs, cats, birds, insects, mice and rats, which carry bacteria on their bodies and in their urine and faeces
- rotting rubbish and waste food
- our clothes and jewellery.

You can prevent the spread of bacteria by having high standards of personal hygiene:

- Wash your hands with soap and water *before* handling food
- Wash your hands with soap and water *after* using the toilet/helping the people you support use the toilet, handling raw food and rubbish, coughing, sneezing, using a handkerchief and touching your skin or hair
- Shower or have a bath every day and keep your clothes clean and tidy
- Keep your nails short and clean and don't wear nail varnish or jewellery
- Keep your hair clean and tied back or covered

- Wear the protective clothing you are given
- Keep wounds covered with coloured waterproof dressings and check that you are allowed to handle food when wearing a dressing
- Do not smoke in a food area – it is against the law!

If you or anyone you live with is unwell, you must tell your line manager. It may be that you will not be allowed to work with food for the time being.

You can prevent the spread of bacteria by having high standards of hygiene in food storage and preparation areas:

- Store raw and cooked food in different fridges. If there is only one fridge, store raw food on the lowest shelves
- Use different work surfaces for preparing raw and cooked food

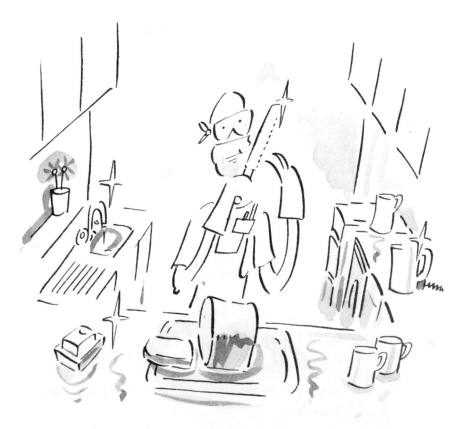

Hygiene is extremely important when preparing food

- Use different equipment, e.g. knives, chopping boards and wiping cloths for raw and cooked food, and store them separately
- Keep work surfaces, equipment and wiping cloths thoroughly clean, especially after using them for raw meat and poultry
- Keep food covered
- Never use food that is past its 'use by' date and bin waste food.

You can prevent the spread of bacteria by avoiding having pets and pests in food storage, preparation and eating areas:

- Check for pets and pests and call the Environmental Health Department for advice if you see signs of an infestation, e.g. droppings
- Throw out any food that might have been spoiled by pets or pests
- Maintain a high standard of cleanliness – sweep floors, wipe up spills, wash and store equipment properly
- Keep doors closed and use fly screens on open windows
- Keep food and waste covered and empty waste bins regularly.

You can also help prevent the spread of bacteria by storing and cooking food at the right temperatures:

- −22°C to 5°C – most bacteria cannot grow at these low temperatures so check that fridges and freezers stay within these limits
- 5°C to 63°C – the Temperature Danger Zone! Most bacteria thrive in the Temperature Danger Zone so store food below 5°C or above 63°C
- 70°C and above – most bacteria are killed at this heat so make sure food is cooked thoroughly and at temperatures above 70°C.

Because body fluids, waste, pressure ulcers, rashes, dressings and soiled linen can cause cross-infection, you must wear protective clothing, such as aprons and gloves, every time your work brings you into contact with them. Good practice means you should also wash your hands thoroughly before and after working with them and wear fresh gloves, aprons or overalls for every person you work with. Ideally, protective clothing should be disposable.

You will read how to wash your hands thoroughly shortly.

DEVELOP GOOD WORK PRACTICE

3.1.3

ACTIVITY 25

Ask your line manager to monitor your ability to use your organisation's health and safety policies and procedures and to sign the Witness Statement to indicate your competence.

Witness Statement

_____ (name of worker)

knows how to apply the organisations policies and procedures in relation to health and safety in their work setting(s) and with the individual(s) they support.

_____ (name of line manager)

_____ (signature of line manager)

_____ (date)

Please give details of the policies and procedures the worker knows how to apply:

Please give details of the setting(s) in which the worker works:

Please give details of the service user group with which the worker works:

3.1.4 Know what you are <u>not</u> allowed to do at this stage of your training in relation to health and safety in your work setting(s) and the individual(s) you support

During the first few months of your employment, you will be required to attend training in, for example, health and safety, COSHH and food hygiene. You read earlier that one of your responsibilities under the HASWA is to only carry out activities that you have been trained to do. Doing work for which you have received no training risks the health and safety of yourself, your colleagues and the people you support.

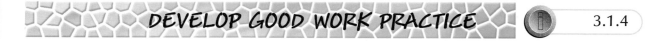

DEVELOP GOOD WORK PRACTICE　　3.1.4

ACTIVITY 26

1 Make a list of the work activities that you are not allowed to do at present.

2 Explain why you are not allowed to carry out these activities.

3.2 MOVING AND HANDLING

About one in three injuries at work are caused by moving and handling, e.g. carrying, pushing, lifting or lowering an object. An object can be a cup of tea; it can also be someone you support. About half of moving and handling injuries affect the back, causing pain, slipped discs, even paralysis. Care workers are more likely to be involved in moving and handling than most other workers, so you can see how risky your job is!

This section aims to raise your awareness of the risks related to moving and handling and the techniques you should use to avoid injuries.

3.2.1 Be aware of key legislation that governs all moving and handling tasks

The purpose of moving and handling law is to prevent moving and handling injuries. There are a number of laws and regulations that tell us how to prevent moving and handling injuries at work.

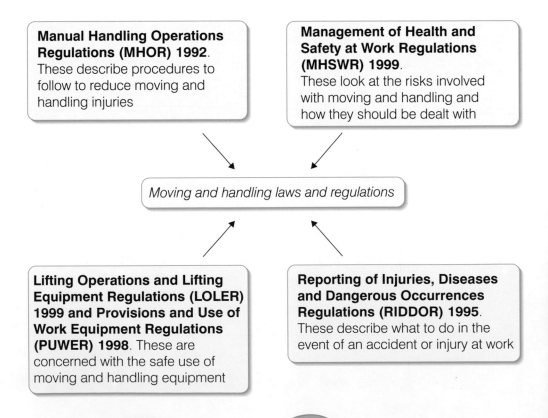

Manual Handling Operations Regulations (MHOR) 1992. These describe procedures to follow to reduce moving and handling injuries

Management of Health and Safety at Work Regulations (MHSWR) 1999. These look at the risks involved with moving and handling and how they should be dealt with

Moving and handling laws and regulations

Lifting Operations and Lifting Equipment Regulations (LOLER) 1999 and Provisions and Use of Work Equipment Regulations (PUWER) 1998. These are concerned with the safe use of moving and handling equipment

Reporting of Injuries, Diseases and Dangerous Occurrences Regulations (RIDDOR) 1995. These describe what to do in the event of an accident or injury at work

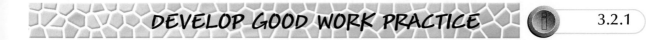

DEVELOP GOOD WORK PRACTICE

3.2.1

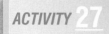

Read your organisation's policy on moving and handling and make a list of the moving and handling regulations that influence the way you do your work.

3.2.2 Know how to assess risks in relation to moving and handling people and/or objects

A moving and handling risk assessment is a check to see:

- how objects are currently moved and handled
- whether the way they are moved and handled can be changed to make it safer.

There are five stages to a risk assessment:

1 First of all, the person doing the risk assessment will ask, 'Is this moving and handling activity risky in any way?' The Health and Safety Executive (HSE) have published a set of guidelines that can be used to help decide whether an activity is risky or not.

2 If they think that the activity is risky, they will then ask, 'Who might be harmed and how?'

3 Next, they will decide whether to get rid of the activity altogether or to change it to one that is less harmful. This is called 'controlling the risks'.

4 They will then write a record that lets people know that the activity has been assessed for risks and how it must be carried out in the future so that it is as safe as possible.

5 Finally, they will set a date to review the risk assessment, i.e. check that the new way of doing the activity is safer or whether it needs further changes.

Risk assessments are common sense procedures but they are very important if moving and handling injuries are to be prevented. All moving and handling activities in your workplace will have been 'risk-assessed' and it is your responsibility to carry them out as the risk assessment tells you.

You should also be prepared to respond to fresh and unexpected risks, such as unpredicted movements made by the person you are supporting, unforeseen breakdowns in equipment and unanticipated changes in the working environment. Unexpected risks can make activities difficult and threaten the health and safety of everyone concerned. For this reason, you should always:

- carry out your own risk assessment prior to doing an activity
- be on your guard for unexpected risks while doing the activity
- report any unexpected risks to your line manager so that they can review the risk assessment.

CHECK YOUR UNDERSTANDING

3.2.2

ACTIVITY 28

Imagine that you have been asked to carry out a risk assessment on a moving and handling activity. In your own words, describe what you would do.

3.2.3 Know safe moving and handling techniques in relation to people and/or objects

Before you are allowed to move and handle objects, including the people you support, you will need to have attended a practical moving and handling training session (see Activity 29).

There are five steps to **SAFER** moving and handling:

1 **S**top and think. Should you be carrying out this moving and handling activity? Can you avoid it at all?

2 **A**ssess the situation. If you cannot avoid the activity, you must follow the procedure given in the risk assessment. But, because situations are never quite as they should be, think about your situation before you start the activity. Do you need to get help from a colleague, to use any equipment or to improve the space you are working in? If the object is a person, can they be encouraged to help you by moving more independently?

3 **F**ormulate an action plan. Once you have assessed your situation you can plan how you are going to carry out the activity.

4 **E**xecute or carry out your plan. When carrying out a moving and handling activity, move your body in a smooth and co-ordinated way:

- *Feet* – Keep your feet as close to the object as possible, slightly apart and with one just in front of the other
- *Knees* – Bend your knees and hips slightly
- *Back* – Stand close to the object and maintain an S-shaped posture; don't twist to lift from the side or stoop to lift from in front; when pushing, lean slightly into the object, and when pulling, lean slightly away
- *Arms and hands* – Use your arms to keep the object close to your body; keep your elbows bent and tucked in to your side; and use your hands, not your fingers, to grasp your load
- *Head* – Keep your chin raised and look straight ahead.

If you are working with a colleague, designate one person to lead the move, e.g. to call out '1, 2, 3 pull!'

5 **R**eview the way you carried out the activity. Did things go to plan? If not, why not? How can you change the activity to reduce the effort and discomfort for all concerned?

By following these five steps to SAFER moving and handling you can maintain your personal health and safety as well as that of your colleagues and the people you support.

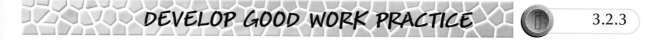

DEVELOP GOOD WORK PRACTICE   3.2.3

ACTIVITY 29

Complete the following details:

1 The Moving and Handling training I attended took place on

_____

2 My Moving and Handling Certificate can be found in

_____

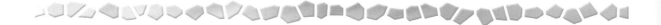

3.2.4 Know what you are <u>not</u> allowed to do in relation to moving and handling at this stage of your training

You may not yet have attended training in moving and handling or been trained in the use of moving and handling equipment. In order to avoid accidents and injuries and to comply with the law, it is most important that you know what you cannot do as regards moving and handling activities.

ACTIVITY 30

> ### CASE STUDY: *Jane*
>
> *Jane has just started a job as a care worker. Many of the people she supports have mobility problems. Some are overweight, some are very frail. Some spend most of their time in bed, others in their chairs.*

Jane has not yet had any training in moving and handling, nor in the use of moving and handling equipment. What activities should she not carry out in relation to moving and handling?

3.3 FIRE SAFETY

3.3.1 Understand how to promote fire safety in your work setting

Although most fires can be prevented, they kill hundreds of people every year.

Ways to prevent fires from spreading include:

- using fire-proof furnishings and bedding – check the labels!
- keeping windows and doors closed. Fire doors must always be kept closed

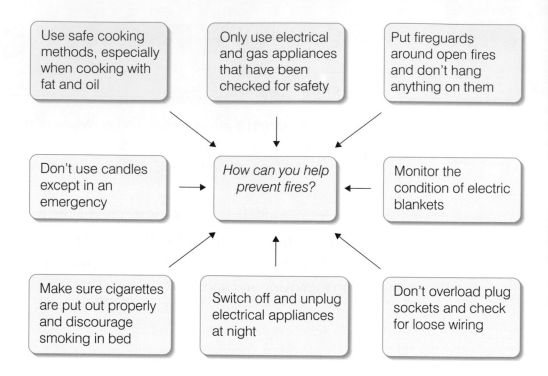

- using smoke alarms. Some smoke alarms have flashing lights or vibrating pads and so are useful for people who have difficulty hearing or seeing. Because smoke alarms are powered by batteries, the batteries need to be checked regularly
- using sprinklers, i.e. water sprays fitted to the ceiling which respond automatically to a fire.

Your organisation's fire safety procedures are based on the Fire Precautions (Workplace) Regulations 1997. All workplaces are different because they are built differently and have different types of people working and living in them. For this reason all workplaces have different fire safety procedures.

It is very important that you know your organisation's procedures for fire safety and that you attend fire safety training at least once a year. However, here is a general checklist:

- If you discover a fire, raise the alarm. Use the fire alarm or simply shout 'Fire!' If you are asked to call the emergency services, dial 999, ask for

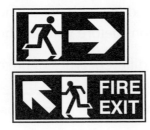
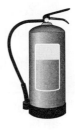

Fire safety signs and equipment

the fire service and describe clearly where the fire is. Don't hang up until the address has been repeated back to you

- Close windows and doors to prevent fire and smoke spreading
- If the people you support can move, help them to a part of the building that is safe or to the assembly point outside. Always use the fire exits and fire escape route
- If the people you support have mobility problems or are ill in bed, it might be more sensible for them to remain where they are and be rescued by the fire service
- Close doors as you pass through them, don't stop for any reason and don't use the lifts
- Be calm, don't panic and don't rush
- Once you have reached the assembly point, check that everyone is accounted for. The fire service will need to know where everyone is
- Don't return to the building until the fire service gives the OK.

Fire blankets and fire extinguishers can be helpful in an emergency, but it is very important to know how and when to use them. Only use equipment before the fire starts to spread. Before tackling a fire, make sure that everyone is outside and that your escape route is clear. If you are not sure what to do, don't take risks – call the fire service.

Fire blankets are used for smothering flames on solids, liquids and chip pans and for wrapping around someone whose clothes are on fire. Check that they conform to British Standard 6575 and read the instructions before you attempt to use them.

Your workplace may be fitted out with fire extinguishers. As with fire blankets, read the instructions before you use them.

The table below describes different types of fire extinguishers.

Contents	Types of fire they can be used for	How they work	How to use them
Dry powder	Most kinds	The powder 'knocks down' the flames	Aim the jet at the base of the flames and sweep it from side to side
Water	Solids only. Never use water on electrical fires or burning fat or oil	The water cools the burning material	Aim the jet at the base of the flames and move it over the area of the fire
Foam or AFF	Foam has limited uses but AFF is effective on most fires except electrical and chip pan fires	The foam forms a blanket or film on the surface of the fire, cutting off the oxygen which 'feeds' a fire	For solids, aim the jet at the base of the flames and move it over the area of the fire. For liquids, aim it at a vertical surface or, if the fire is in a container, at the inside edge of the container.

It is very helpful for the people you support to know your organisation's fire safety procedures. You can teach them about fire safety by:

- explaining the meaning of different alarms and fire safety signs, e.g. fire alarm signs, signs for fire exits and escape routes. If you work with people who have a sight or hearing impairment, your workplace should have adapted signs and alarms, e.g. signs in Braille, flashing lights, vibrating buttons. Make sure everyone knows what these mean

- inviting fire fighters in to talk about fire prevention, and showing videos and having discussions about what to do in the event of a fire

- having regular fire drills to make sure that everyone recognises the fire alarm, knows how to walk away from a fire without panicking and knows how to help others who are confused or have mobility problems.

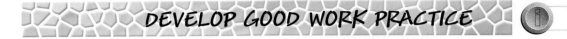

DEVELOP GOOD WORK PRACTICE

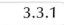 3.3.1

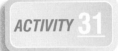

Complete the following details:

1 The Fire Safety training I attended took place on

_____

2 My Fire Safety Certificate can be found in

_____

3.4 EMERGENCY FIRST AID

Your workplace's procedures for dealing with first aid emergencies are based on the Health and Safety (First Aid) Regulations 1981. It is very important that you know and follow these procedures and that you attend first aid training and refresher courses on a regular basis.

3.4.1 Know what to do in response to illness or accident

Primary health care services are provided by GPs (General Practitioners), nurses, dentists, opticians and pharmacists. These are the people we go to first in the event of ill health.

GPs diagnose and treat illnesses, prescribe medicines, give advice and refer patients on to specialist consultants if necessary. They also carry out minor surgery. If someone you support becomes ill, you need to telephone their GP. If you are unsure about the seriousness of their illness, there may be an NHS Drop In Centre nearby where you can take them for advice or treatment. You could also telephone NHS Direct and talk your concerns through with an expert.

If someone you support has an accident, they may require first aid. First aid is a skill that requires training and practice. The aims of first aid are to:

- **p**reserve a casualty's life
- **p**revent further harm
- **p**romote (help) their recovery.

If you haven't yet attended first aid training, you shouldn't attempt to give anything more than the basic first aid described below. If you have been on an Emergency First Aid or Appointed Person's First Aid course in a previous job or at school or college and your certificate is up-to-date, you may be competent (skilled) in giving artificial ventilation and cardio-pulmonary resuscitation (CPR). However, only give first aid that you know you can do safely and with confidence.

Basic first aid for emergencies – **DR ABC**

D IS FOR DANGER

Before giving help of any kind, check the situation for danger to yourself. Don't attempt to help if helping would put you in danger. Don't delay in sending someone to get qualified help (see below).

R IS FOR RESPONSE

Try to get a response from the casualty. Talk to them and gently shake their shoulders. If they are conscious and respond to you in a normal way, reassure them that help is on its way. Move them to a safer place if there is a risk of further injury. If they don't respond, continue to talk to them and to gently shake their shoulders. Check that qualified help is on its way.

A IS FOR AIRWAY

If the casualty is unconscious or responds to you with difficulty, your priority is to check that their airway – mouth and throat – is not blocked. A blocked airway leads to choking and suffocation. If you can, remove the cause of the blockage, taking care not to push it further down the throat. Open the airway by tilting the casualty's head backwards and lifting their chin. Check that qualified help is on its way.

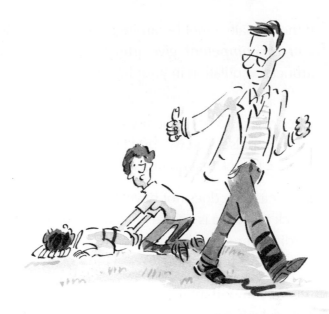

If you are unable to give first aid safely, ask someone to fetch help

B IS FOR BREATHING

Check that the casualty is breathing. You can do this by putting your cheek close to their mouth and feeling for their breath, and by looking down over their chest, watching for breathing movements. If they are breathing, put them into the recovery position. This keeps the airway open. You will practise putting someone into the recovery position in your first aid course. Check that qualified help is on its way.

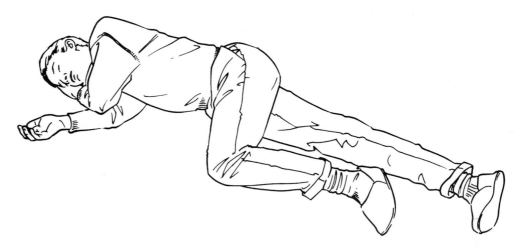

The recovery position ensures that the casualty's airway is open

If the casualty is not breathing, check that qualified help is on the way. *If you are competent*, give artificial ventilation. You will learn how to give artificial ventilation in your first aid course.

C IS FOR CIRCULATION

Check whether the casualty's heart is beating. You can do this by feeling for their pulse. You will practise checking for a pulse in your first aid course. Check that qualified help is on its way.

If the casualty does not have a pulse or a heartbeat (cardiac arrest), check that help is on the way. *If you are competent* give cardiopulmonary resuscitation (CPR). You will learn how to give CPR in your first aid course.

It is very important that you only give first aid that you know you can do safely. If you are not competent, confident and qualified you can make things worse for the casualty. If you are not sure what to do, send for someone who is competent and help them in whatever way they ask.

If there is a first aid emergency, dial 999 for an ambulance. When you dial 999 it is important that you are able to answer clearly and calmly questions about:

- the casualty, such as their name and age
- the location of the emergency – the address and telephone number
- the cause of the emergency
- what first aid has already been given.

CHECK YOUR UNDERSTANDING

3.4.1

ACTIVITY 32

1 Ned has fallen and is lying in the road. You talk to him and he responds in a normal way. What should you do?

2 Mrs P stumbles and falls as she gets up from the table. You talk to her but she has difficulty speaking and seems to be gasping for air. What should you do?

3 Sally has fallen down the stairs. She does not respond to you when you talk to her. What should you do?

▲▲▲▲▲▲▲▲▲▲▲▲▲▲▲▲▲▲▲▲▲▲▲▲▲▲▲▲▲▲▲▲▲▲▲▲

3.4.2 Understand basic emergency first aid techniques

The following first aid techniques are basic and common sense. However, once you have given help you should still summon support from a competent person.

Minor wounds and bleeding	Wash your hands. Tie a clean dressing (from the first aid box if possible) firmly over the wound. If the bleeding continues, put another dressing on top of the first one and get help
Suspected broken bones (fractures)	Don't move the casualty unless they are in a dangerous position. Get help
Burns and scalds	Cool with cold water. Get help
Eye injuries	Wash your hands. Wash the casualty's eye with clean, cool water. Don't attempt to remove anything from the eye. Get help

You will learn how to deal with severe bleeding, more complicated wounds, broken bones and serious burns and scalds in your Emergency First Aid or Appointed Person's First Aid course.

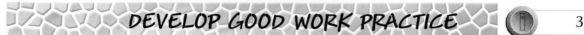

DEVELOP GOOD WORK PRACTICE   3.4.3

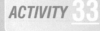

ACTIVITY 33

Complete the following details:

- The Emergency First Aid/Appointed Person's First Aid training I attended took place on _____

- My Certificate can be found in _____

- What first aid are you allowed to give now?

  _____

- What first aid are you not allowed to give?

  _____

- Why aren't you allowed to give anything more than basic first aid?

  _____

3.5   INFECTION PREVENTION AND CONTROL

The people you support may be ill, old or disabled in some way; or they may live in unhealthy surroundings. Because of this, they are at risk of catching infectious diseases. Your workplace will have procedures for making sure that infection is prevented and controlled. It is very important that you know and follow these procedures and that you attend infection control training.

3.5.1 Understand the main routes of infection

The table below gives some examples of infectious diseases and how they are caused.

Infectious diseases	Causes
Sore throats, boils, pneumonia, tuberculosis (TB), tetanus, impetigo, gastroenteritis, MRSA	Bacteria
Influenza (flu), colds, mumps, herpes (e.g. cold sores), AIDS, hepatitis B	Viruses
Thrush (*Candida*), ringworm	Fungi
Infestations	Animals such as lice and mites

What are the main routes of infection, i.e. how do bacteria, viruses, fungi and animals get into the body?

- *Through the skin*. Diseases caught by direct contact (being touched by an infected person) and indirect contact (touching things like handkerchiefs and towels that an infected person has used) include scabies, ringworm, impetigo and herpes.
- *Through the airways*. Inhaling (breathing in) the droplets sprayed out when an infected person coughs or sneezes can cause, e.g. colds, influenza (flu) and measles; and inhaling infected dust can cause tetanus.
- *Through the digestive tract*. As you read above, eating food and drink that has been contaminated can cause food poisoning.
- *Through the use of health care instruments*. For example, using needles after they have been used on an infected person can cause AIDS and hepatitis B.

CHECK YOUR UNDERSTANDING

3.5.1

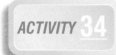

Find out what infectious diseases are experienced by the people you support. Produce an information sheet that describes what causes them and how they get into the body.

3.5.2 Know how to prevent the spread of infection

Infection can be prevented from spreading in a number of ways. The most important way is to help the people you support stay healthy by making sure that they eat well, are immunised against infectious diseases such as flu, and that they take their medication as prescribed.

You can also help prevent the spread of infection by following workplace procedures and manufacturer's instructions, for example when you are:

- working with service users who have particular types of infectious disease
- cleaning, disinfecting and sterilising equipment
- cleaning up spillages and dealing with waste.

Another very important method of preventing the spread of infection is to:

- wash your hands with soap and water **before**
  - handling food
  - giving medication
  - giving first aid and handling wounds
- wash your hands with soap and water **after**
  - using the toilet and helping others to use the toilet
  - coughing, sneezing, using a handkerchief and touching skin, hair, dentures
  - giving first aid and handling wounds
  - making beds

- handling raw food and rubbish
- handling equipment, laundry and waste contaminated with body fluids.

You will learn how to wash your hands effectively shortly.

As you read earlier, protective clothing is important because it prevents cross-infection, i.e. it prevents you from being infected by the people you support and prevents them from being infected by you. Therefore, you must wear the protective clothing your organisation gives you. In addition, any equipment you use in an infectious situation must be sterile and either disposed of or re-sterilised after use.

Finally, you can help prevent the spread of infection by following RIDDOR procedures for reporting infectious diseases that occur in your work setting. Once an infectious disease has been reported, measures can be put into place to prevent it spreading by nursing the infected people in isolation (barrier nursing), isolating very vulnerable people who are at risk of catching the infection (reverse barrier nursing), developing and giving vaccinations, and so on.

CHECK YOUR UNDERSTANDING   3.5.2

ACTIVITY 35

Look back at the infectious diseases you identified for your answer to Activity 34. Include in your information sheet how these diseases can be prevented.

3.5.3 Know how to wash hands properly

Effective handwashing is the **nationally recognised way to prevent the spread of infection.**

You must learn and practise the correct technique for washing your hands:

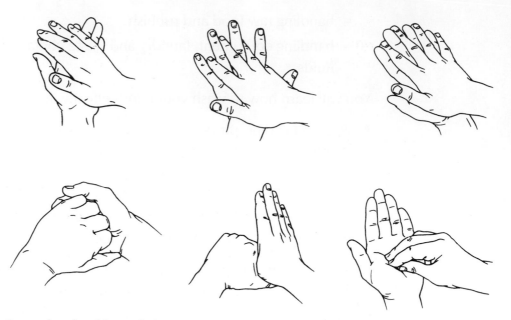

Correct handwashing technique

1 Wet your hands with hot running water and rub some soap between your palms

2 Rub your right palm over the back of your left hand and then your left palm over the back of your right hand

3 Rub your palms together again but this time with your fingers interlocked

4 Rub the back of the fingers of your left hand with your right palm and then the back of the fingers of your right hand with your left palm

5 Rub around your left thumb with your right palm and then around your right thumb with your left palm

6 Rub your left fingertips round and round in your right palm then your right fingertips round and round in your left palm

7 Rub your left wrist with your right hand then your right wrist with your left hand

8 Rinse both hands thoroughly under running water and dry them carefully on clean paper towels

You should wash your hands even if you have been wearing gloves.

Sometimes there will not be a sink where you can wash your hands, in which case you should use a handrub. Handrubs, like sinks, should be near the place where you carry out your activities – too far away means your hands will keep hold of bacteria and infection may spread.

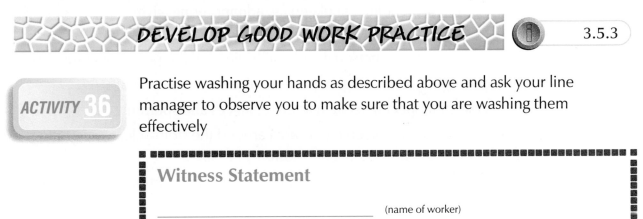

DEVELOP GOOD WORK PRACTICE

3.5.3

ACTIVITY 36

Practise washing your hands as described above and ask your line manager to observe you to make sure that you are washing them effectively

Witness Statement

_____ (name of worker)

knows how to wash their hands properly.

_____ (name of line manager)

_____ (signature of line manager)

_____ (date)

3.6 MEDICAL AND HEALTH CARE PROCEDURES

3.6.1 Understand your organisation's policies and procedures in relation to medication and health care tasks

Medication can be abused, i.e. taken for no clinical reason; it can be misused, sometimes with horrific consequences, as in the case of Dr Harold Shipman; and it can have harmful side-effects such as dizziness, tiredness, headache and nausea. Health care activities can cause distress, embarrassment and put physical health at risk. For these reasons, organisations that provide caring services must have special arrangements in place in relation to medication and health care tasks.

You may be required to carry out the following medication and health care tasks in your work with the people you support:

- recording, handling, safekeeping, administering (giving) and disposing of medicines
- maintaining the personal and oral hygiene of the people you support
- preventing and caring for pressure ulcers
- collecting specimens such as urine, faeces and sputum
- colostomy care (keeping the area around the stoma clean, and fitting, changing and disposing of colostomy bags)
- catheter care (ensuring the genitals are clean, insertion and withdrawal of the catheter and collection of urine)
- PEG feeding, which includes keeping the area around the PEG clean, keeping the PEG clean and free from blockages, and giving feeds
- giving injections.

Your organisation will have policies and procedures in place that aim to protect the health and safety of the people you support in relation to medication and health care tasks.

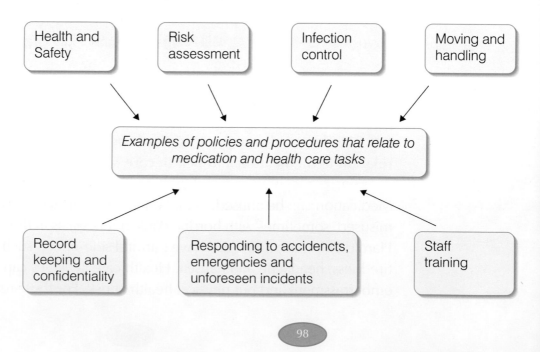

CHECK YOUR UNDERSTANDING   3.6.1

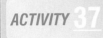

Find out what medication and health care tasks you will be required to carry out and describe the policies and procedures that govern how you should do them.

3.6.2 Understand how to apply your organisation's policies and procedures in relation to the individuals you support

Health and safety

You read about your health and safety responsibilities earlier. These apply to medication and health care tasks as much as to the rest of your work.

Risk assessment

The people you support must, if they have the ability, be given the opportunity to carry out their own health care procedures. They must be given the opportunity to self-administer, i.e. to keep and take their medicine themselves. They must also be allowed to refuse medication. Refusing to take medication can put their and other people's health and safety at risk. Your role is to provide them with the information they need in order to be able to make an informed decision, which in turn protects people's right to health and safety.

If someone you support does not <u>consent</u> to take their medication, you must not deceive them by, for example, disguising it in their food and drink. Make your line manager aware of the situation without delay. Similarly, make sure that any problems (such as in swallowing tablets) are reported to your line manager without delay.

Infection control

You must:

- wear appropriate protective clothing
- use sterile equipment when appropriate, e.g. syringes
- keep equipment such as medicine trolleys, medicine pots, spoons, drinking glasses and water jugs scrupulously clean
- wash your hands thoroughly both before and after giving medication and carrying out health care tasks.

Control of substances that are hazardous to health

You must follow COSHH procedures when:

- working with body waste and fluids as they are likely to be infectious
- administering medicines – abuse or deliberate misuse of medication is against the law; accidental misuse can be fatal
- disposing of health care equipment such as soiled linen and sharps. Like body fluids and waste, they can spread infections. Sharps also present a risk of injury.

Moving and handling

You must follow safe moving and handling procedures, for example to prevent accidents, injuries and pressure ulcers from developing or becoming worse.

Record keeping and confidentiality

A record must be kept of all:

- medicines brought into the care home or the person's own home
- medicines that people take – most organisations record these details in Medical Administration Records (MARs)
- medicines that are disposed of – it is best practice to return unused and out-of-date medication to the pharmacy

- health care activities – most organisations record these details in care plans
- specimens taken and the results of tests.

Records relating to the people you support must remain confidential.

Responding to accidents, emergencies and unforeseen incidents

Situations such as when the wrong dose of a medication has been given (e.g. a tablet that should be given every 12 hours is given every 4 hours) or medication is given to the wrong person must be reported and recorded straightaway. Similarly, if someone's behaviour or condition changes as a result of taking medication or receiving health care, you must report and record your observations without delay.

Staff training

In order to carry out medication and health care tasks, care workers *must* be trained and be able to demonstrate competence.

In addition, you must use the principles of care and the Codes of Practice in your work in order to support people's independence, maintain their privacy and dignity, and promote their choice to be cared for in the way that meets their preferences, wishes and needs.

DEVELOP GOOD WORK PRACTICE   3.6.2

ACTIVITY 38

Ask your line manager to check that you have an understanding of how to use medication and health care policies and procedures and to sign the Witness Statement to confirm your understanding.

Witness Statement

_____ (name of worker)

understands how to apply medication and health care policies and procedures in relation to tasks to the individual's they support.

Witness Statement *(continued)*

_____ (name of line manager)

_____ (signature of line manager)

_____ (date)

Please give details of the medication and health care tasks that the worker understands how to apply:

```
[                                                    ]
```

3.6.3 Know what you are <u>not</u> allowed to do in relation to medication and health care procedures at this stage of your training

You read earlier that before they can carry out medication and health care tasks, care workers *must* be trained and able to demonstrate competence.

CHECK YOUR UNDERSTANDING   3.6.3

ACTIVITY 39

1 Describe what medication and health care tasks you are not allowed to do at this stage in your training and explain why not.

```
[                                                    ]
```

2 What training will you need to undergo in order to be able to carry out medication and health care tasks?

3.7 SECURITY

Feeling secure means feeling safe and feeling safe is important for good health and well being. This section aims to raise your awareness of security measures and how you can minimise risks to your safety and well being and the security of the people you support.

3.7.1 Be aware of security measures in your workplace

The people you support have a need and a right to feel safe and secure. For this reason, your workplace will have various security measures in place to protect them from danger and harm.

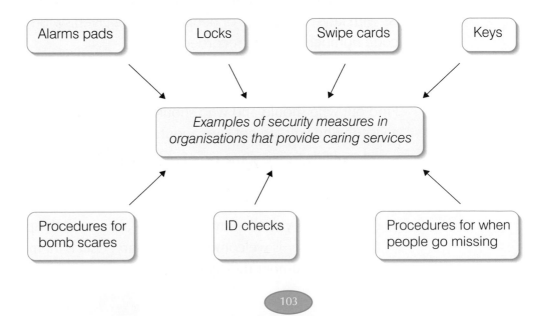

Alarms

There are many types of alarm, including:

- personal alarms and alarms sited in central areas and used in the event of, for example, intruders or people behaving in a challenging way
- security alarm systems, which are triggered by people approaching doors or windows or entering a building without permission.

Your role is to know how to use alarms at work, not to deal with security emergencies.

Locks

Locks are put in place to make sure that certain areas in a building can only be accessed by authorised people. Most organisations have a named key holder who is responsible for:

- the safe-keeping of keys
- issuing keys to authorised people
- maintaining a signed record of the people who borrow keys
- ensuring that keys are returned for safe-keeping after use
- making sure that keys are not copied.

Some organisations use swipe cards and key pads as alternatives to locks and keys. Swipe cards allow authorised people access to buildings; punching a code number into key pads opens locks on gates, doors, etc. As with keys, the names of people who are given swipe cards and key pad code numbers must be recorded.

Checking the identity of visitors

Find out who should and who should not be in your workplace. If there is a visitor who you are not sure about:

- ask politely to see some proof of identity, such as an ID badge, a driving licence that has a photograph or the telephone number of the organisation they represent
- confirm with your line manager, colleagues and the people you support that the visitor is welcome – if necessary, check them out using the telephone number they gave you

- give them a name badge and make sure they complete the visitors book on arrival and when they leave.

Missing people

Because care workers don't have eyes in the backs of their heads, sometimes the people they support can go missing. On such occasions, you must follow your organisation's Missing Person's procedure, which will tell you to:

- inform your manager as soon as you discover someone is missing
- inform the police if you think the missing person is capable of leaving the building (be prepared to describe them in as much detail as you can)
- make a thorough search of the building, including all the obvious places as well as under beds, in cupboards, and so on
- go out and look for the person if you have been given permission. If you know them well, you are likely to have some idea of where they might have gone.

Bomb scares

It is unlikely that you will be involved in a bomb scare; however, you must be prepared. Your organisation will have procedures for dealing with bomb scares made by telephone but in general:

- take the caller seriously
- encourage them to give you as much information as possible and make a note of what they tell you
- inform your line manager and the police straightaway
- start the evacuation procedure.

If you receive a bomb threat in the post or notice a suspicious package, follow your organisation's reporting and evacuation procedures. Keep any letters and envelopes that arrive in the post in good condition as the police will need them for evidence. Never attempt to deal with a suspicious package yourself.

Make sure you attend bomb scare and evacuation training and always follow your organisation's bomb scare procedures.

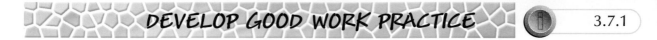

DEVELOP GOOD WORK PRACTICE 3.7.1

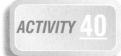

ACTIVITY 40 Find out about the security systems that are in place where you work. Produce an information leaflet for staff and the people you support that describes how the systems work and explains why they are necessary.

3.7.2 Recognise the risks to your personal safety and well being in your work setting(s) and the safeguards required to minimise these

The people you support can put your health and safety at risk by behaving in challenging, sometimes violent ways. Reasons why people become violent include:

- their state of health, which can be very stressful and traumatic
- loss of independence, which can be frustrating
- dementia, which causes a loss of social skills, confusion and inappropriate behaviour
- mental health problems or learning difficulties, which can prevent people understanding what's going on, making them feel scared and threatened.

In order to protect yourself from violence, you need to know who can become violent, the sorts of situations that can lead to violence and how to reduce the dangers. Talking to colleagues and reading individual care plans will enable you to anticipate and prevent problems or deal with them before they get out of hand.

Another situation which could put you at risk is when you are working alone. Even though you are part of a care team, there may be times when you will be on your own, for example at night or when you are transporting money.

Working without your colleagues close-by can knock your self-confidence. Because they are not there to support you, you might start to feel isolated and to wonder whether you are doing your job correctly. The solution to this problem is to make sure you are well trained and practiced in giving care. You should also know who to contact if you get into difficulty.

Working alone can make you vulnerable. For example, you might be accused of doing something you have not done. If you can demonstrate that you are always conscientious and that you follow work procedures carefully, you and those you have to report to will be confident that you have done your job properly.

Make sure your line manager knows where you are and what you are doing at all times. This is particularly important when you are working alone. It means that you can be traced if you get lost, your car breaks down or you are late arriving at work.

A checklist for minimising risks to your personal safety and well being:

- be trained for the different situations you may have to face
- follow work procedures at all times
- be able to make contact with your colleagues or line manager, e.g. carry a mobile phone or a pager
- never be afraid to ask how to deal with a situation.

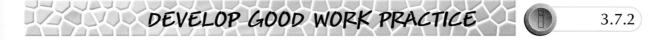

DEVELOP GOOD WORK PRACTICE   3.7.2

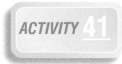

ACTIVITY 41 Tell your line manager about the risks to your personal safety and well being at work and how you can minimise them and ask him or her to sign the Witness Statement to confirm your understanding.

Witness Statement

_____ (name of worker)

recognises the risks to their personal safety and well being in their work setting(s) and the safeguards required to minimise them.

_____ (name of line manager)

_____ (signature of line manager)

_____ (date)

Please give details of the risks to personal safety and well being to which the worker is exposed:

Please give details of the safeguards required to minimise these risks:

Communicate effectively

The ability to communicate is very important. It allows us to interact with other people and form relationships with them. And because care work goes hand-in-hand with the development of good relationships with the people you support, effective communication is a skill you need to develop as a care worker. This chapter aims to help you develop your communication skills and to show you how you can encourage the people you support to communicate with you.

Successful completion of the activities in this chapter will enable you to demonstrate your understanding of the Common Induction Standard *Communicate effectively*. It will also give you an opportunity to develop evidence for key skills unit Communication at level 1.

What is covered in this chapter?

This chapter contributes to the knowledge and understanding you need for the following NVQ Care units at level 2:

HSC 21 : Communicate with, and complete records for individuals

HSC 22 : Support the health and safety of yourself and individuals

HSC 24 : Ensure your own actions support the care, protection and well being of individuals

4.1 ENCOURAGE COMMUNICATION

4.1.1 Know what motivates people to communicate

The people you support have a right to be heard but may find it difficult to communicate, for example they may speak another language, have a hearing impairment, be ill or distressed. However, to do your job properly you need to know how they feel, what they want and need and if they have any concerns. So you need them to communicate with you.

How can you motivate people to communicate with you? Active support encourages communication, and the following section describes ways in which you can provide active support.

Show respect for people's individuality, life histories, cultural backgrounds and rights, and challenge other people whose behaviour is discriminatory or unfair. Discrimination and behaviour that does not value equality and diversity does not motivate communication.

Show that you are interested in what people are trying to communicate by:

- using active listening and appropriate verbal communication and body language. You will learn about these shortly
- not interrupting and giving them sufficient time. Learn to respect silences – they give people an opportunity to think about what they want to say and to reflect on what they have heard
- using their preferred means of communication. Find out how they want to communicate by asking them (they are the experts!) and others who know and understand them. Be prepared to adapt the way you communicate to meet their needs by using their <u>first language</u>, writing, signing, lip reading, pictures, <u>interpreters</u> and so on
- checking that you have understood each other. Repeat back what you think you have heard as this gives them an opportunity to check that you have understood them correctly and ask questions to check that they have understood you.

Show respect for their privacy and be discreet when completing their records and sharing information about them with others. This will help them put their trust in you and feel able to talk to you in confidence.

Show that you are interested in the factors that affect their ability to communicate, and that you know what to do if you notice any changes in their ability to communicate. You will learn about barriers to communication shortly.

Be professional in the way you work, by following the communication instructions written into care plans and by using the principles of care when communicating and completing records and reports.

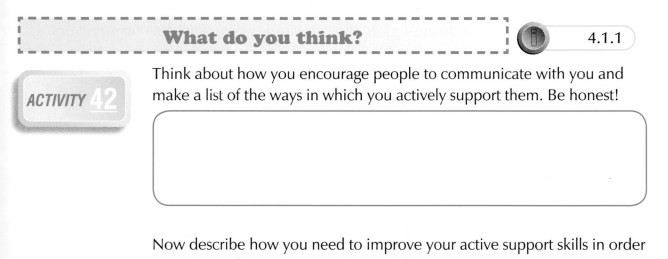

What do you think?

4.1.1

ACTIVITY 42

Think about how you encourage people to communicate with you and make a list of the ways in which you actively support them. Be honest!

Now describe how you need to improve your active support skills in order to motivate them to communicate with you.

Why do you need to make these changes in your behaviour?

4.1.2 Recognise the main barriers to communication

Communication is difficult when there are barriers that prevent people from understanding each other.

> ### CASE STUDY: *Grace*
>
> *Grace is at the Health Centre with her residential care worker, waiting to see the doctor. She is very worried about her health. The waiting room is hot, stuffy and gloomy. It is also noisy because of telephones, the traffic outside and chatter from the office.*
>
> *The receptionist calls Grace to the desk and asks her a string of questions, using lots of medical expressions. The receptionist is from another country – neither Grace nor her care worker recognise the accent – and seems to be quite stressed.*

Do you think that the receptionist would succeed in obtaining the information she needs from Grace? Not likely – the situation is loaded with communication barriers!

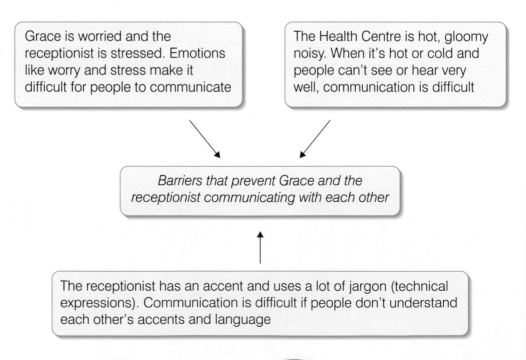

Grace is worried and the receptionist is stressed. Emotions like worry and stress make it difficult for people to communicate

The Health Centre is hot, gloomy noisy. When it's hot or cold and people can't see or hear very well, communication is difficult

Barriers that prevent Grace and the receptionist communicating with each other

The receptionist has an accent and uses a lot of jargon (technical expressions). Communication is difficult if people don't understand each other's accents and language

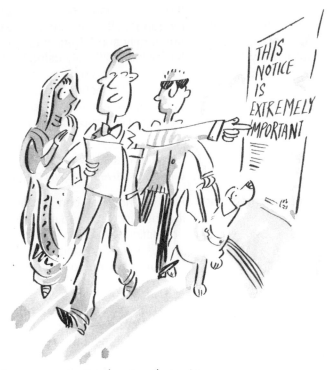

Be aware of the communication barriers that exist

This sort of situation is quite common so it is no wonder that there are breakdowns in communication! But you need the people you support to communicate with you, so it is your responsibility to:

- be alert to barriers that make it difficult for them to communicate
- play your part in making things easier for them by overcoming barriers.

The table below describes examples of communication barriers and how you can help overcome them for the people you support.

Communication barriers	How you can help
Emotional difficulties, e.g. stress and anxiety; and mental health problems such as dementia and depression	Make sure you provide a safe and private environment, be patient, reassure the person that you are interested in what they want to say; use your listening skills (see below)
Physical health problems and disabilities, e.g. stutter, stroke	Again, be patient, reassure the person that you are interested in what they want to say; use your listening skills

continued

Language differences and difficulties using and understanding speech, e.g. because of learning difficulties or cerebral palsy	If possible, learn and use the person's preferred spoken language; alternatively, get help from colleagues, their friends and family and others who can act as interpreters or translators. If they have difficulty using or understanding spoken language, you could use signs, symbols, pictures, writing, objects of reference, technological aids such as voice-recognition computer software and specialist equipment that meets their individual communication needs
Jargon, slang and accents that are difficult to understand	Explain what the words and expressions mean or, better still, use alternatives that will be understood
An uncomfortable environment and sensory impairments	Find out how you can improve lighting and heating and check that hearing aids and glasses are in working order. If the person has difficulty hearing you could get help from a signer or learn and use the sign language they are familiar with. If they have difficulty hearing you could help them to communicate through touch
Cultural differences that affect the way people communicate, e.g. personal space differences, how people like to be addressed and whether they are allowed to talk to someone of the opposite sex	Find out how someone's cultural background affects the way they communicate and make sure you communicate with them in ways that meet their cultural needs

Don't forget that the problem could be you! Make sure that your behaviour does not block communication. The next section looks at behaviour as a form of communication.

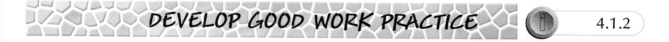

DEVELOP GOOD WORK PRACTICE   4.1.2

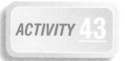

ACTIVITY 43

Find out from two or three of the people you support about difficulties they have when communicating with you and your colleagues. Jot down what they tell you and make notes on how you can help overcome these barriers.

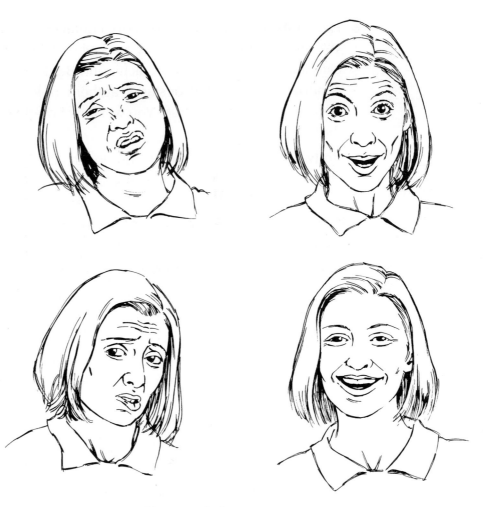

Facial expressions can reveal how you feel

4.1.3 Understand how behaviour is a form of communication

Body language is a very important aspect of communication – it tells people how we feel, something which words on their own aren't very good at. A positive use of body language encourages communication.

Body language takes a number of forms:

- **Facial expressions**, e.g. smiles, frowns, looks of amazement and disgust. Looking interested and reflecting back (mirroring) people's facial expressions shows that you understand how they feel and encourages them to communicate with you.

- **Eye contact** Appropriate use of eye contact lets someone know that you are interested in what they are saying; and gazing into their eyes can be a sign of a romantic attachment! But looking out of the window while they talk or staring at them for long periods does not encourage communication. You will look bored and could make them anxious.

- **Body posture and position** If you slouch or turn away while someone is talking to you, you will look fed up and uninterested. On the other hand, leaning slightly towards them in an upright but comfortable position shows that you are giving them your full attention.

- **Body movements or gestures** Tapping your foot or fingers while someone is talking to you is a sure sign that you are bored, perhaps in a hurry and don't want to listen. On the other hand, nodding your head shows that you are trying to understand what they are saying and moving your hands gives expression to what you are saying.

- **Dress** The way you dress says a great deal about you. It tells people who you are, what your job is, and whether you have power or influence over them. So be aware of the effect you can have on people if, for example, you wear a uniform, a mask or an apron.

- **Proximity or closeness** Being physically close to someone can be a useful way of showing that you want them to tell you how they feel. But beware – you must respect their 'personal space' and not enter it without permission.

- **Touch** You will read about the use of touch to promote communication shortly.

- **Paralanguage** This is to do with the way we say things. When we are sad or depressed, we tend to speak quietly, slowly, on a low note and without much variation in our tone of voice. But when we are pleased, excited or anxious we speak more loudly and quickly, with ups and downs in our tone of voice. Mirroring the way people say things when we talk to them shows that we understand how they feel and encourages them to communicate.

Sometimes people's body language can become upsetting and disruptive. We call this 'challenging behaviour'. Challenging behaviour can be spoken, using a threatening tone of voice or speaking loudly and very quickly; it can also be physical, e.g. an aggressive posture, hostile gestures and prolonged eye contact. The people you support may behave in challenging ways for a number of reasons, for example they may:

- be distressed because of ill health
- be stressed because of noise or relationship problems
- have a low opinion of themselves because they are losing their independence
- not recognise that their behaviour is 'out of line' because they are confused or on medication that has changed their behaviour.

It is important to respect people's right to choose how to behave but it is equally important that they behave in ways that do not put other people's health, safety and well being at risk. If someone starts behaving in a challenging way, try to calm things down. Use words, body language and a tone of voice that are friendly and non-hostile. Don't try to invade their space or restrain them but give them a firm explanation of why their behaviour is unacceptable. If things become violent and unsafe, your priority is to call for help and to get yourself and others out of danger. Don't try to deal with violent situations until you have more experience.

Your organisation will have procedures that describe how to deal with incidents of challenging behaviour, including how you should report and record them. There are training courses that you can attend, which will help you develop the skills needed for dealing with challenging behaviour. Find out when you can attend one.

CHECK YOUR UNDERSTANDING

4.1.3

ACTIVITY 44

1 Observe and make a note of the body language used by your colleagues and the people they support when communicating with each other.

2 Explain why they used these methods of behaviour.

4.2 USE COMMUNICATION TECHNIQUES

4.2.1 Understand the basic forms of verbal/non-verbal communication and how to use these in your work setting(s)

In situations where speech or verbal communication is possible, only about 10% of the communication is spoken. The other 90% is non-verbal communication or body language. You read about the different forms of body language in the previous section and the following diagram summarises how you should use body language in your work with the people you support.

As people need to see your body language to fully understand what you are communicating, make sure that the lighting is neither too bright nor too dim.

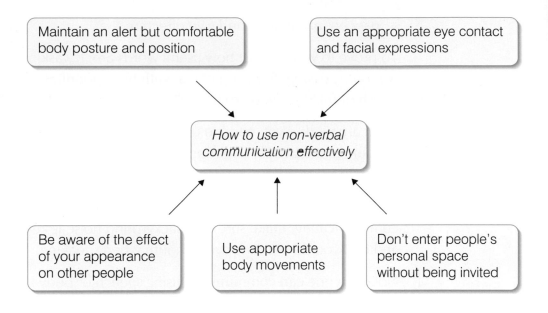

Maintain an alert but comfortable body posture and position

Use an appropriate eye contact and facial expressions

How to use non-verbal communication effectively

Be aware of the effect of your appearance on other people

Use appropriate body movements

Don't enter people's personal space without being invited

Although it only makes up a small part of a communication, verbal communication is very useful! It allows us to:

- let others know how we feel and what we want
- find out about things, by asking questions

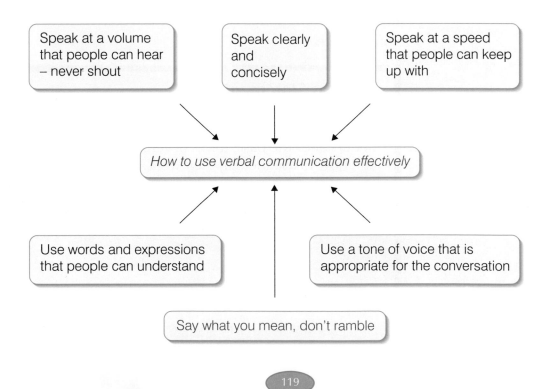

Speak at a volume that people can hear – never shout

Speak clearly and concisely

Speak at a speed that people can keep up with

How to use verbal communication effectively

Use words and expressions that people can understand

Use a tone of voice that is appropriate for the conversation

Say what you mean, don't ramble

- pass on information and give directions.

To prove to yourself just how useful words are, try asking someone, *without speaking*, for a cup of tea, with two spoonfuls of sugar and a splash of milk! It's good to talk!

As a care worker you need to use verbal communication effectively to encourage the people you support to communicate and to make yourself understood.

Because people need to hear you to fully understand what you are communicating, make sure that background noise is kept to a minimum and that you do not cover your mouth when speaking.

Not everyone can communicate using speech or body language. You read about alternative communication techniques earlier.

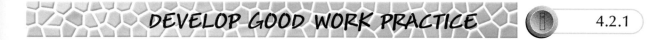

DEVELOP GOOD WORK PRACTICE   4.2.1

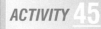

ACTIVITY 45

Ask your line manager to check your understanding of the basic forms of verbal and non-verbal communication, to monitor your ability to use them effectively, and to sign the Witness Statement to indicate your competence.

Witness Statement

_____ (name of worker)

understands the basic forms of verbal and non-verbal communication and how to use them in their work.

_____ (name of line manager)

_____ (signature of line manager)

_____ (date)

4.2.2 Understand how to listen effectively

There is little point encouraging the people you work with to communicate with you if you don't listen to what they tell you! For this reason it is important that you develop effective listening skills.

> **CASE STUDY: *Mr Simpson***
>
> *Mr Simpson used to be quite chatty but recently has become very quiet, preferring to sit alone; and he looks troubled.*

Your line manager has asked you to spend some time with Mr Simpson, to find out what's troubling him. How would you encourage him to talk to you about the way he feels?

You already know that appropriate body language shows you are paying attention and are interested in what you are being told. So, as a good listener you would:

- look at Mr Simpson as you and he chat together
- sit in a relaxed position, perhaps leaning slightly forward to help you concentrate on what he tells you
- change your tone of voice and the expression on your face to mirror his feelings.

You could also encourage him to continue by nodding your head and making noises like 'yes' and 'mmm'.

Effective listeners do more than just hear words and recognise feelings. They also 'read between the lines' or 'hear' what isn't said. In this way they get a full understanding of what is being communicated. We call this 'active listening'.

> **CASE STUDY: *Mr Simpson (continued)***
>
> *Mr Simpson tells you that his daughter is having problems at home and does not have time to visit him any more.*

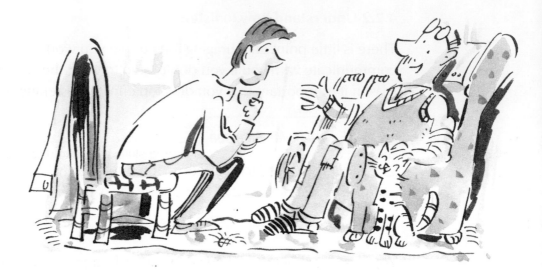

A good listener makes service users feel comfortable in expressing their feelings and concerns

'Reading between the lines', what do you think Mr Simpson is saying? Perhaps that in addition to being worried about his daughter, he is missing her visits and becoming lonely and depressed?

As a good listener you will pick up on things that are not actually said but it is important to check that your understanding is correct. Don't assume that what you have 'heard' is correct. The way we 'hear' things can change depending on the way we feel. For example, do you hear things in the same way when you are busy and stressed as when you are relaxed and have lots of time to spare? Check your understanding by asking questions that give people the chance to express themselves more clearly.

The point about being a good listener is that, by showing interest and trying to understand what you are being told, the people you support will feel valued and be encouraged to tell you more. The more you know, the better you will be able work with them and do your job.

What do you think?

ACTIVITY 46

Ask your colleagues or your line manager for feedback on your listening skills. Make a list of the skills you use now and another list of those you need to develop.

Listening skills I use now	Listening skills I need to develop

4.2.3 Understand how to use touch to promote communication

To touch and be touched meets a basic human need. We need to touch others to communicate our feelings for them and we need to be touched to know that we are accepted, loved, and cared for. In addition, a cuddle or a massage can be calming, relaxing and improve our well being. A congratulatory hand shake and a pat on the back can raise our self-confidence and feelings of self-worth.

A great deal of what you do as a care worker involves the use of touch, for example when you give:

- emotional support, e.g. stroking someone's hand, giving them a hug, signalling your presence by a touch on their shoulder if they have a sensory impairment

- physical support and protection, e.g. guiding people who have poor sight, supporting people who have mobility problems or who are at risk of falling, carrying out moving and handling activities
- support with day-to-day living activities such as eating and drinking and the more intimate activities of bathing, using the toilet, getting dressed, shaving and so on.

If used appropriately, touch can show the people you support that you are genuinely concerned for them and their well being, which in turn encourages them to communicate with you.

4.2.4 Understand when touch is not appropriate

Not everybody is comfortable with being touched. Imagine that you have become quite dependent and need to live in a residential care home. How would you feel if you had to have your bottom wiped by someone you don't know very well? How would you feel if your religion says that only close relatives are allowed to touch you? How would you feel if you were abused as a child yet have to be undressed and bathed by someone else? You might feel uncomfortable, embarrassed or scared.

These sorts of feelings inhibit (prevent) communication between people. So when you carry out activities that involve the use of touch it is very important that:

- you have the person's permission to touch them
- you let them guide you in the way you carry out the activity
- you work in a professional way, using the principles of care and following the GSCC Code of Practice
- your attitude ensures that they are completely at ease with everything you do and that they maintain their dignity and feel confident, safe and secure.

You learned earlier that it is important not to restrain people who behave in challenging ways. Holding someone down can aggravate the situation, putting health and safety further at risk. If someone is in danger of harming themselves or others, or of damaging property, your line manager will

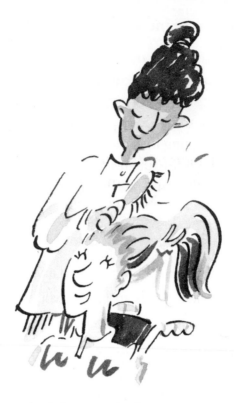

Touch is an important method of communication

make the decision about whether or not it is appropriate to use physical restraint. If you are not able to calm a situation through the use of the non-hostile means described above, seek help without delay.

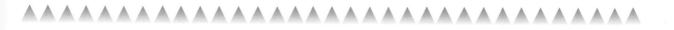

CHECK YOUR UNDERSTANDING   4.2.3/4

ACTIVITY 47

Write an anonymous case study of one of the people you support that describes:

- the physical contact you have with them and how you use it to encourage them to communicate with you
- when and why you wouldn't use physical contact with them.

4.3 The principles of good record keeping

4.3.1 Know the use and purpose of each record or report the worker has to use or contribute to

Records and reports play a very important role in care work. Using records and reporting information enables you and your colleagues to work in a way that is lawful and effective and that protects the rights and promotes the health, safety and well being of the people you support.

Different organisations have different names for records and reports, some of which are described below, but their purpose remains the same.

Care plans are used to record and report:

- people's needs and how, when and by whom their needs are to be met
- the caring activities you carry out
- any problems you have carrying out your activities and what you do about them
- observations you make that could indicate a change in someone's condition and care needs.

Recording and reporting your observations and any problems you have paves the way for a care plan review so that people's needs can continue to be met effectively.

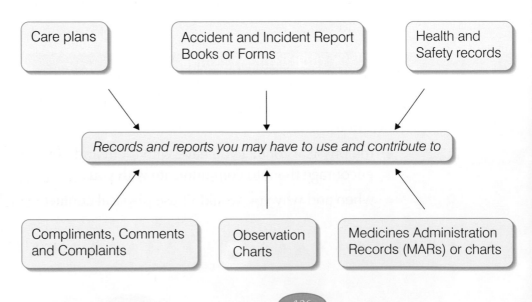

Accident and Incident Report Books or Forms are used to record and report:

- accidents, emergencies and dangerous incidents. Reporting and recording, e.g. slips and trips, episodes of choking and challenging behaviour means that steps can be taken to prevent them happening again

- the activities you carry out as a result of an accident, emergency or dangerous incident.

Details of accidents, emergencies and incidents are needed by the emergency services in the event that they become involved, and by insurance companies in the event that a claim is made.

Health and Safety records and risk assessments are used to record and report:

- health and safety hazards, such as those caused by people's behaviour, the appliances and equipment you use, the building you work in and security issues. Reporting hazards means they can be dealt with before an accident or incident happens

- the activities you must carry out to protect people from danger, harm and abuse. But remember – you must only do activities for which you have been trained

- anything you need to make your work more safe. Your employer is responsible for making sure you can work in a safe and healthy way.

Compliments, comments and complaints. Complaints and comments made about your organisation give your employer an opportunity to review and improve the way services are provided. Complaints and comments made about you give you an opportunity to:

- think about your attitude and the way you carry out your activities

- change the way you work and improve your relationships.

Complaints and comments should therefore be seen as positive feedback. Encourage and help the people you support to use complaints and comments procedures. Similarly, encourage and accept praise and kind words and use them to demonstrate your professional development. You will read about professional development in Chapter 6.

Observation charts are used to record routine measurements such as weight change, body temperature, blood pressure, pulse rate, food and fluid intake, the quantity of urine passed, and skin colour and condition. Observation charts enable health professionals to diagnose and treat medical conditions.

Medicines Administration Records (MARs) or charts. When you have been trained you may be involved in administering medication. Medicines Administration Records (MARs) or charts are legal documents which provide evidence that the people you support have been given their medicines according to the prescription. They tell you:

- which medicines are prescribed for each person
- when they must be given
- what the dose is
- any special information, e.g. medical and cultural requirements and personal preferences regarding what, when and how to take medicines.

MARs or charts must be completed every time medicine is given. They must show exactly what medicines were given, when medicines were not given or were refused, and they must be signed and dated.

CHECK YOUR UNDERSTANDING

4.3.1

ACTIVITY 48

Complete the table to show your understanding of the purpose of records and reports that you use or contribute to and who might want or need to read them.

Records or reports I use/contribute to	Purpose of these records and reports

4.3.2 Know how to record information that is understandable, relevant to purpose, clear and concise, factual and checkable

It is extremely important that any information you record or that someone records on your behalf is clear and understandable. It is equally important that any information that you record on tape is audible and capable of being heard clearly and understood.

Consider the following telephone message.

<u>Telephone message</u>
Mrs H rang the bell isn't working today there's a chap coming.
Bill

Although we can read what Bill has written, can we understand it? Did Mrs H use the telephone to ring in to work or did she ring the bell? Is it Mrs H or the bell that isn't working? Is the chap coming today, is Mrs H not working today or is it the bell that's not working today? And when is 'today'? – there's no date. All very confusing!

Information you record must also be concise and relevant, i.e. it must get to the point quickly and only include what is important.

<u>Observation record</u>
Food intake
Mr J didn't eat much breakfast this morning. He ate some of the egg but none of the bread and he left his cup of tea on the bedside table. It was cold. When I went to collect his tray he was watching the TV. There was a programme on about gardening and he told me he used to enjoy working on his allotment. He used to grow his own vegetables and sell them when he had too many for his own use.
P. White 1st April 10am

Although this record is clear and understandable, it rambles on and much of what is said isn't relevant to a record of food intake. Records that aren't concise are frustrating to read; and irrelevant information is a waste of time, both for the person recording the information and for the person who has to read it.

Because records are used to monitor people's needs, they must be factual, i.e. accurate, and they must be checkable. Express the facts exactly as you saw them:

- don't make anything up
- never give your opinions, feelings or thoughts
- don't exaggerate anything
- don't leave anything out because, for example, you are in a hurry.

What do you think is wrong with this entry in a care plan?

<u>Care Plan</u>
1 April
Dorothy was a bit of a pain this evening. She had a right old moan at me when I took her in her bedtime drink. She's got another bruise on her arm. Fallen over again I suppose.
Wendy, 9pm

First of all, how do you think Dorothy would feel if she discovered she had been described as a 'bit of a pain' and as having 'had a right old moan'? Annoyed? Insulted? Remarks like these are subjective, i.e. one person's point of view. They are not necessarily how somebody else might describe Dorothy's behaviour and so are not factual.

Secondly, had Dorothy really fallen over? This remark may well be true but it should be checked before being put in writing.

The entry in Dorothy's care plan should have been written like this:

<u>Care Plan</u>

1 April

Dorothy wasn't very happy this evening, especially when I gave her some hot milk. She has a bruise on her arm. Please investigate:

1 If there is something concerning her.
2 Whether she would prefer an alternative to hot milk at bedtime.
3 Whether she has had a fall.

Wendy, 9pm

To sum up, records must be:

- clear (easy to read or hear)
- easy to understand
- concise (short and to the point)
- relevant (contain only important information)
- factual (accurate and objective)
- checkable.

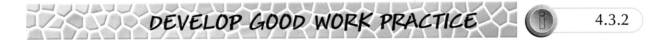

DEVELOP GOOD WORK PRACTICE   4.3.2

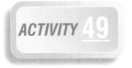

ACTIVITY 49

Just about everybody needs to improve their record making skills! Talk with your line manager about the records that you write (or that someone writes on your behalf) or make using tape. Tick the boxes to show which skills you are good at and which skills you need to improve.

Records I make:	I'm good at this	I need to improve this
are easy to read		
are easy to understand		
are concise and to the point		
include only relevant information		
include only factual information		
include information that can be checked		

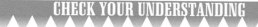

4.3.3 Understand the importance of, and your role in, record keeping

CHECK YOUR UNDERSTANDING

4.3.3

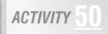

ACTIVITY 50

You read earlier about the importance of keeping records. Produce a poster for your staffroom that:

- lists the different types of records that care workers use or contribute to. You may have to use or contribute to records that were not described earlier (be sure to describe all the records you use or contribute to)
- describes your role in keeping these records
- explains why it is important to keep these records.

4.3.4 Understand how to use reports and records appropriately

Before you use records and reports containing personal information, you must get permission from the appropriate people, e.g. the people you support and your line manager.

Follow your organisation's confidentiality and security procedures and protect people's right to privacy when:

- getting records and reports out of storage. Let someone in authority know if you have any difficulty accessing records and reports
- using records and reports to guide you in your work
- updating records and reports. As you know, you need to complete records and reports accurately and in ways that can be understood by others who need to use them. Let someone in authority know if you have any difficulty updating records and reports
- returning records and reports to storage.

When you have updated their records and reports help the people you support to understand:

- why and what you have reported and recorded
- why you need to share the information with others and who you need to share it with.

Finally, make sure you follow your organisation's procedures for passing information on to appropriate people.

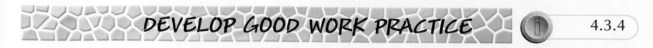

DEVELOP GOOD WORK PRACTICE

4.3.4

ACTIVITY 51

Ask your line manager to monitor your ability to use reports and records appropriately and to sign the Witness Statement to indicate your competence.

Witness Statement

_____ (name of worker)

understands how to use reports and records appropriately

_____ (name of line manager)

_____ (signature of line manager)

_____ (date)

Please give details of records and reports that the worker has to use:

5 Recognise and respond to abuse and neglect

Care workers need to be able to recognise when the people they support are neglecting themselves and when they are being abused or neglected by others. They also need to know how to deal with abuse and neglect. This chapter aims to give you an understanding of the signs and symptoms of abuse and neglect and of how to respond to situations where you think abuse and neglect may be taking place. It builds on what you have learnt about the principles of care, effective communication and your role as a worker.

Successful completion of the activities in this chapter will enable you to demonstrate your understanding of the Common Induction Standard *Recognise and respond to abuse and neglect*. It will also give you an opportunity to develop evidence for key skills unit Communication at level I.

What is covered in this chapter?

This chapter contributes to the knowledge and understanding you need for the following NVQ Care units at level 2:
HSC 24 : Ensure your own actions support the care, protection and well being of individuals

5.1 LEGISLATION, POLICIES AND PROCEDURES

5.1.1 Be aware of key legislation in relation to abuse and neglect

Abuse is cruel behaviour that is usually carried out on purpose by the abuser so that he or she can be seen to be powerful and 'in charge'. Abusive behaviour is humiliating and degrading and has disturbing and long-lasting effects on people's health and well being. Neglect, which means failing to care for others, and self-neglect, which means failing to care for ourselves, are usually not deliberate but can have similar disturbing and long-lasting effects.

Some of the people you support are particularly vulnerable to abuse and neglect because they are weak and defenceless. You have only to read the newspapers and watch the television to realise how frequently people who use caring services, such as older people, children and people with learning difficulties, are abused and neglected.

Everyone has the right to live their life free from abuse and neglect. The Human Rights Act 1998 protects everyone's rights to freedom from humiliating and degrading treatment. It is a very important piece of legislation to organisations that provide social care because it underpins the way that care is given to vulnerable people.

The Care Standards Act 2000 is also important to organisations that provide social care. It requires employers and care workers to meet National Minimum Standards of conduct; and it requires the Commission for Social Care Inspection (CSCI) to inspect care homes, to check that they are meeting the Standards.

National Minimum Standard 18 for work in care homes for older people tells us that residents must be protected from deliberate or unintentional abuse and neglect, and inhuman or degrading treatment. It also says that procedures must be in place for:

- responding to suspicion or evidence of abuse or neglect, including whistle blowing, which you will read about shortly
- following up accusations and incidents of abuse without delay and recording any action that is taken

- making sure that abusive behaviour is dealt with appropriately. You read about this in Chapter 5
- protecting residents' money, valuables and financial affairs.

The Care Standards Act also states that care workers cannot start work until they have been checked against the Protection of Vulnerable Adults (POVA) list. The POVA list identifies people who may be unsuitable to work with children or other vulnerable members of society. POVA checks are part of a Criminal Records Bureau (CRB) Disclosure or check.

If an organisation needs to take on new staff quickly they can ask for a POVA First check. The POVA First check confirms whether potential workers are not on the POVA list and can start work before having a full CRB check. All existing care home staff must have a satisfactory CRB check to continue in their jobs. The Commission for Social Care Inspection also inspects care homes to make sure that all staff have satisfactory POVA and CRB checks.

The Care Standards Act and the Care Homes Regulations 2001 aim to ensure that the health and welfare of residents is protected by requiring staff to be trained in the prevention of abuse and neglect. As discrimination is a form of abuse, the various discrimination laws that you learnt about in Chapter 1 are important in protecting people from inhuman or degrading treatment.

The Children Act 2004 is aimed at keeping children safe and healthy. It is the law that shapes *Every Child Matters: Change for Children*, the programme responsible for children's services.

CHECK YOUR UNDERSTANDING

5.1.1

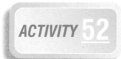

Find out what legislation covers your role in preventing abuse and neglect and say why it is important.

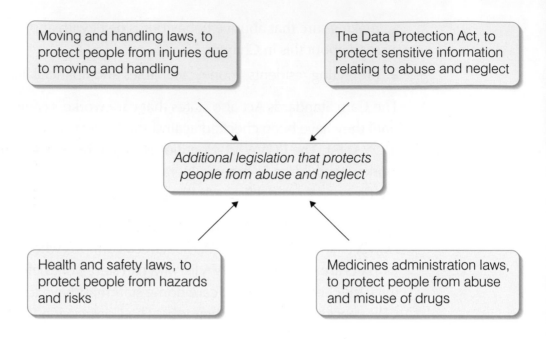

5.1.2, 5.1.3 Understand and know how to apply your organisation's policies and procedures in relation to abuse and neglect

As you know, policies and procedures are based on legislation. The way you do your work is also governed by the principles of care and the GSCC Code of Practice (see Chapter 2). Abuse and neglect happen when care workers do not follow policies and procedures, the Code of Conduct or use the principles of care in their work.

The table below gives some examples of policies and procedures that are related to abuse and neglect and shows how they link to legislation and the Code of Practice. To obey the law and maintain safe standards of care in your work, you must follow your organisation's procedures in relation to abuse and neglect. As you read earlier, if you make mistakes because you do not follow procedures correctly, you can be held legally responsible.

Examples of key legislation and Codes of Practice in relation to abuse and neglect	Linked policies and procedures
Health and Safety and Moving and Handling regulations	Risk assessment, COSHH, Infection Control, Moving and Handling policies and procedures, etc., which protect the people you support from abuse and neglect caused by accidents, challenging behaviour, prolonged exposure to urine, rough handling and so on
The GSCC Code of Practice that covers people's rights to take risks	How to promote people's right to deal with risks to their health and well being themselves
The Care Standards Act, Health and Safety and Anti-discriminatory regulations, and the Code of Practice that covers dealing with discriminatory, abusive behaviour and neglect	The action to take when you observe discriminatory behaviour; how to respond to situations and behaviour so that you avoid further risk to yourself and others; and how to report suspected abuse and neglect
The Care Standards Act that covers meeting people's changing needs and the Data Protection Act that requires records to remain confidential except in special circumstances	How to record and report, in confidence, changes in people's condition that you think are related to abuse and neglect
The Code of Practice that states that you must not abuse the trust of the people you support	How to make sure that people feel able to discuss, in confidence, their care and other people's behaviour toward them
The Code of Practice that states that you must communicate in an appropriate, open, accurate and straightforward way; and the Data Protection Act that requires reports to be made in confidence	How to let people know your role in protecting them from abuse and neglect; and how to let them know your responsibility for disclosing, in confidence, what you are told in relation to abuse and neglect
Medicines Administration regulations	How to prevent the misuse or abuse of drugs

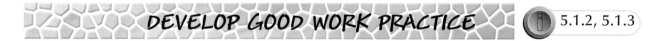

DEVELOP GOOD WORK PRACTICE 5.1.2, 5.1.3

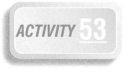

ACTIVITY 53

Ask your line manager to check your understanding of your organisation's policies and procedures in relation to abuse and neglect, to monitor your ability to use them, and to sign the Witness Statement to indicate your competence.

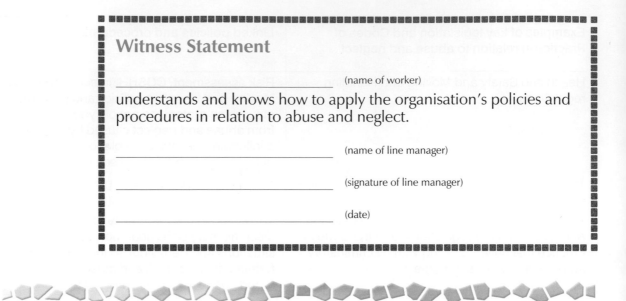

Witness Statement

_____ (name of worker)

understands and knows how to apply the organisation's policies and procedures in relation to abuse and neglect.

_____ (name of line manager)

_____ (signature of line manager)

_____ (date)

5.2 UNDERSTAND THE NATURE OF ABUSE AND NEGLECT

5.2.1 Know what the following terms mean: physical, sexual, emotional, financial and institutional abuse; and self-neglect and neglect by others

Many of the people you support are particularly at risk of abuse or self-abuse because they are unable to defend themselves against an abuser or their own behaviour. Self-abuse can be a way of coping with emotions – it is a way of making emotional pain into something physical that can be seen by others. This section describes the different types of abuse that you need to be familiar with.

Physical abuse is behaviour that causes physical pain or injury.

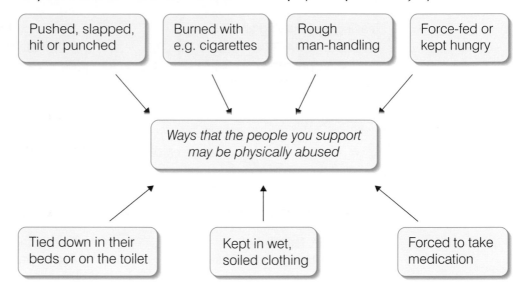

Sexual abuse is unwanted, illegal sexual behaviour.

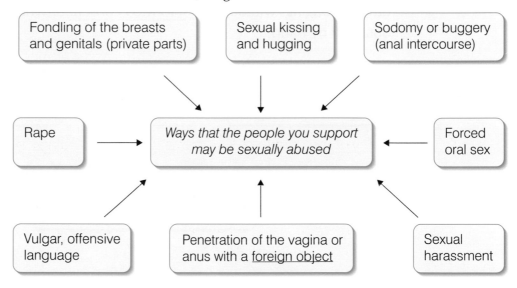

Emotional abuse is behaviour that hurts or injures people's feelings.

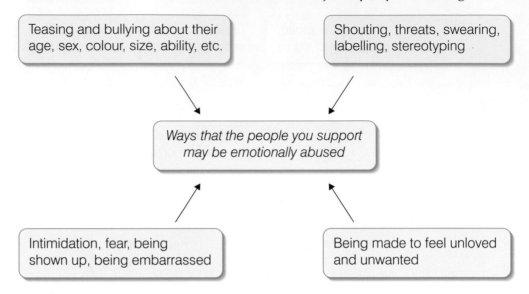

Financial abuse is the illegal use of someone's property, money and other belongings without their <u>informed consent</u> or where their consent is obtained by <u>fraud</u>.

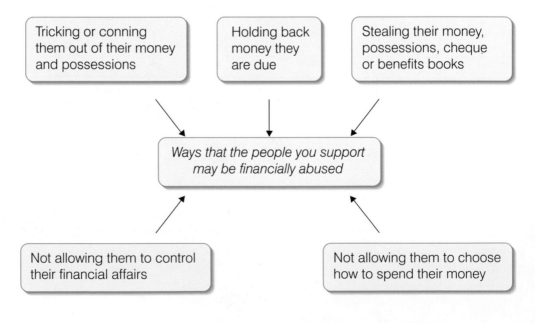

Institutional abuse is where an institution's work procedures and routines become more important than the people needing support.

Controlling the way they live, e.g. meals, medication and toileting have to be carried out at certain times

Taking away their independence because it's easier and quicker for staff to do everything

Ways that institutions may abuse the people you support

Not allowing them to take part in or make contributions to the running of the organisation that provides their care

Treating everyone the same because there isn't time to get to know people as individuals

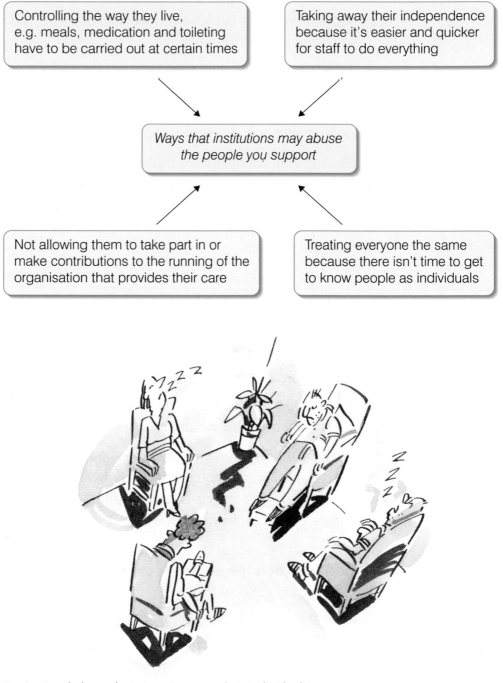

Institutional abuse denies service users their individuality

Self-neglect, as you read above, means failing to care for ourselves. We all tend to neglect ourselves from time to time, for example how often have you:

- skipped breakfast because you went to bed late, didn't hear the alarm and were pushed for time?
- spent your last few pounds on treating the children when you needed spoiling more than they did?
- forgot to make or keep an appointment with the dentist because looking after everybody else seemed more important?

Neglecting yourself by, for example, not getting enough rest, not looking after yourself emotionally and not eating properly will, in due course, have an effect on your health and well being. Unless you find time to care for yourself, you will become rundown and no longer able to care for others, never mind yourself.

Many of the people you support may neglect themselves, for example by:

- not taking their medication
- not eating and drinking properly
- not caring for their personal hygiene and appearance
- not looking after their own comfort
- not staying in touch with friends and family
- not letting you know what they want and how they feel.

There are lots of reasons why people neglect themselves. They may be depressed and have no interest in looking after themselves; they may find it physically difficult to look after themselves; and they may have forgotten how to care for themselves. But whatever the reason, self-neglect is a form of abuse.

Neglect by others. Neglecting or failing to care for others is also a form of abuse. Are you guilty of neglecting the people you support? For example:

- Do you ever forget to do things, such as take a glass of water to someone who is thirsty because you've got so many other things on your mind?
- Do you ever promise to, for example, help someone go to the toilet, but, because you are so busy, you do not keep your promise?

Although you would never neglect people on purpose, circumstances can mean that it is often all too easy to overlook their requests and needs. But like neglecting yourself, neglecting the care of the people you support can lead to a down-turn in their health and well being. Thirst can quickly become dehydration and urine-soaked clothing can lead to rashes, sores and ulcers in addition to a loss of dignity. You will read more about the signs and symptoms of neglect and self-neglect shortly.

CHECK YOUR UNDERSTANDING

5.2.1

ACTIVITY 54

CASE STUDY: *Pitt Street*

Pitt Street Day Care Centre provides activities, social stimulation and lunch for older people in the community. Some of the staff are not very kind – they get frustrated and use offensive language, they make the elderly people eat food they do not like and they leave them unattended while they have cigarette breaks. Because the centre is understaffed, the elderly people have to wait their turn to go to the toilet and it is not unusual for some of them to have accidents while they are waiting. The younger members of staff find this disgusting and often make the offenders sit in their wet clothing until there is time to deal with the situation. There is always a raffle but sometimes no prize.

List the different types of abuse, neglect and self-neglect that occur at Pitt Street Day Care Centre.

5.3   RECOGNISE THE SIGNS AND SYMPTONS OF ABUSE AND NEGLECT

5.3.1 Recognise the signs and symptoms associated with physical, sexual, emotional, financial and institutional abuse, and neglect by self or others

The damage that abuse and neglect cause to people's health and well being is tragic. Because you have a responsibility to maintain the health, safety and well being of the people you support, you need to know the signs and symptoms of abuse, neglect and self-neglect.

The signs of **physical abuse** include bruises, broken bones, burns and blisters, cuts, finger and restraint marks and pressure ulcers. Physical abuse also affects people's behaviour and mental health. People who experience physical abuse become scared and withdrawn and lose their self-confidence and self-esteem. Some people who have experienced physical abuse become abusers themselves.

People who are **emotionally abused** can feel picked on, frightened and discriminated against. They may stop eating and sleeping properly, become disheartened, lose their self-confidence and self-esteem and become aggressive. Eventually, they find it difficult to show their feelings and build relationships. As a result, they lose their sense of belonging and become withdrawn and lonely.

The signs of **sexual abuse** include bleeding, bruising, swelling, STIs and unwanted pregnancies. Victims of sexual abuse can feel disgusted, humiliated, embarrassed and frightened. They may feel ashamed, degraded and lose their dignity and self-respect. Eventually, they may become withdrawn and unable to develop loving sexual relationships. Some people who have experienced sexual abuse become abusers themselves.

Financial abuse causes worry and upset, depression and a loss of interest in financial affairs. People who are financially abused often become dependent and lose the power to run their lives as they want. And a

146

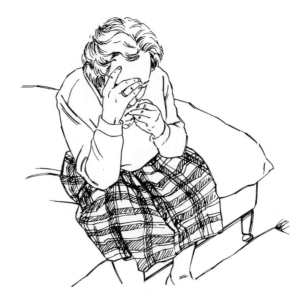

The signs and symptoms of abuse

shortage of money means they are not able to buy themselves a good quality of life, which leads to physical and mental ill health.

Institutional abuse takes away people's ability to make choices, express their views and be independent. As a result, they lose interest in everything around them and become sluggish, bored, depressed, lose their self-worth and may eventually develop feelings of despair and utter hopelessness.

The signs and symptoms of **neglect** and **self-neglect** include:

- a decline in physical and emotional health
- weight loss or gain
- poor personal hygiene
- a grubby, scruffy appearance and living environment
- loneliness
- loss of intellectual skills, e.g. interest, communication and problem-solving skills
- loss of social skills, e.g. the ability to develop and maintain relationships, which can lead to social isolation.

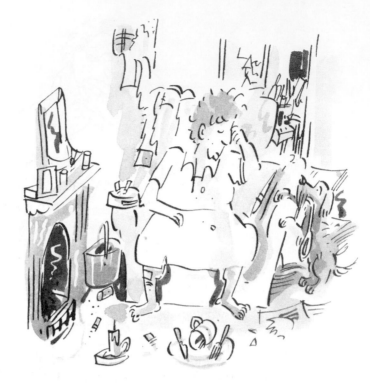

Care workers must look out for signs of self-neglect

ACTIVITY 55

Look back at Activity 54. Describe the signs and symptoms that would alert you to the fact that people at the Pitt Street Day Care Centre were being abused, neglected or were self-neglecting.

5.4 UNDERSTAND HOW TO RESPOND TO SUSPECTED ABUSE AND NEGLECT

5.4.1, 5.4.2 Understand the need to report any suspicions about the abuse or neglect of the individual(s) you support; know when and to whom suspected abuse/neglect should be reported

The people you support may be abused or neglected by members of their family, their friends, carers, care workers, in fact by anyone who has contact with them. It is hard to accept that people who are emotionally close to or who work with people who need support can be abusive or neglectful, but the reality is that some are.

As you read above, abuse and neglect have tragic effects on people, both physically and emotionally. Abuse and neglect by care workers is extremely bad practice and a dismissible offence because it shows that they do not use the principles of care in their work, nor do they follow organisational procedures and the social care Codes of Practice. For example, if you abuse and neglect the people you support, you:

- fail to show them respect
- deny them their right to safety and protection from harm
- take away their dignity.

In addition, abuse and neglect are wrong, unjust, put people's lives in danger and are against the law.

For these reasons you have a responsibility to monitor your own behaviour, to make sure that nothing you do could be seen as abuse or neglect. Check with your colleagues and line manager that your behaviour is always appropriate and get help if you or they are worried about the way you work.

You also have a responsibility to monitor other people's behaviour. You learnt how to deal with challenging behaviour in Chapter 3. If you are worried that one of your colleagues is abusing or neglecting the people you support by, for example:

- hurting them, physically or emotionally
- not responding to their needs
- being rude to them
- not respecting their privacy
- receiving gifts from them or borrowing their money,

talk your concerns over with your line manager without delay.

If you are worried that your line manager is being abusive or neglectful, talk to somebody in a more senior position without delay. But never make accusations about colleagues or people in authority unless you have actually witnessed abuse or neglect or you have evidence to prove your case. There might be a very good explanation for behaviour that appears to be abusive.

If someone you support tells you (discloses) that they are being abused or neglected:

- show them that you believe them – this is most important
- listen to them carefully and check that you have understood them correctly
- ask 'open' questions that help them give you a full description of what happened, e.g. 'Can you tell me what happened?'
- don't ask 'yes/no' questions, e.g. 'Did she hit you?' as these won't give you a full story
- make sure they understand that you will have to tell your line manager what they have told you. Be sensitive in the way you handle this – you need to remain trustworthy

- make sure they understand that other people may have to be told but only those people who are concerned for their safety. Again, be sensitive
- reassure them that anything they say will be treated with respect and confidentiality.

Follow your organisation's procedure for recording and reporting disclosed abuse and neglect. This means:

- reporting your worries, what you have seen and what you have been told to your line manager without delay
- record information in writing as soon as possible, before you forget any details.

Records of abuse and neglect may be read by doctors, the police, social workers and so on. For this reason, what you write, what someone writes on your behalf or what you record on tape must be clear, understandable, relevant, to-the-point, factual and checkable and must follow procedures regarding confidentiality.

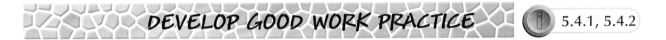

DEVELOP GOOD WORK PRACTICE 5.4.1, 5.4.2

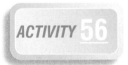
ACTIVITY 56

1 Produce an information sheet for a new colleague that describes why care workers need to report their suspicions relating to abuse and neglect.

2 Read your organisation's procedure for reporting abuse and neglect and use what it tells you to add to your information sheet a description of:

a. when to report concerns about abuse and neglect

b. who to report concerns to.

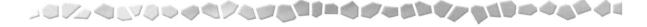

5.4.3 Know what to do if you suspect any *child* is being abused or neglected

Everyone who comes into contact with children has a duty to safeguard and promote their welfare. You may, in the course of your work, come across a child who you suspect is being abused or neglected. The following checklist aims to help you deal with situations like this.

1 Know and follow your organisation's procedures for promoting and protecting children's safety and well being, and know who at work you should report your concerns to.

2 Report your concerns to the relevant person in your organisation. You may be asked to try to find out from the child what has happened. If so, communicate with them in a way that suits their age, understanding and preference. If you are worried about what they tell you, reassure them and maintain their trust but do not promise to keep anything secret.

3 Because accusations of child abuse or neglect may lead to a criminal investigation, do not do anything to put an investigation at risk, for example do not ask the child leading questions, i.e. questions that put ideas into their head; and do not attempt to investigate the accusations yourself.

4 Report your communication with the child to the relevant person in your organisation and make a record of the child's name, address(es), sex, date of birth, the name(s) of their parent(s)/carer(s), your concerns, and the details of your communication with them.

5 Concerns should also be reported to social services or the police. If you have responsibility for making reports to outside agencies like these, be prepared to give the details you recorded (see above), as well as anything else you know about the child, e.g. special needs. It helps to know who to report concerns to – keep a list of the names of people who are responsible for dealing with accusations of abuse and neglect.

ACTIVITY 57

> **CASE STUDY: Gemma**
>
> Gemma is the granddaughter of one of the gentlemen residents at
> Fairways Care Home. She is eight years old. Sue, one of the care
> workers, has recently noticed bruises on Gemma's face, arms and
> legs and finds her increasingly sad, withdrawn and tearful. Sue is
> concerned that Gemma is being physically abused.

What would you advise Sue to do?

5.5 'WHISTLE BLOWING'

A 'whistle blower' is someone who exposes wrong-doing in an
organisation in the hope of stopping it. Whistle blowers usually expose
wrong-doing to the public, e.g. through the media, or to people in
positions of authority. You will read about these shortly.

The Public Interest Disclosure Act 1998 protects whistle blowers from
being discriminated against or dismissed. If a whistle blower does suffer
from discrimination or dismissal as a result of whistle blowing then they
are entitled to make a claim at an employment tribunal.

5.5.1 Understand that your first responsibility is to the safety and well being of the individual(s) you support

Your primary responsibility as a care worker is to protect the safety and
well being of the people you support. You must therefore report any

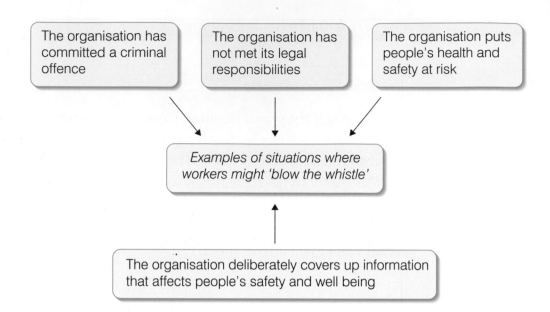

The organisation has committed a criminal offence

The organisation has not met its legal responsibilities

The organisation puts people's health and safety at risk

Examples of situations where workers might 'blow the whistle'

The organisation deliberately covers up information that affects people's safety and well being

concerns you have about abuse and neglect or any situations that might affect your ability to provide safe care. If you feel unable, for whatever reason, to report your concerns to your organisation, or you aren't satisfied that your organisation has dealt with your concerns properly, you may 'blow the whistle'.

CHECK YOUR UNDERSTANDING

5.5.1

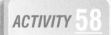

ACTIVITY 58

CASE STUDY: **Mr Brown**

The following case study is based on a true story.

Jacky Smith is the manager of a small care home that supports people who are elderly and disabled. One day, a care worker told Jacky that Mr Brown, the owner of the home, was behaving strangely in one of the rooms. When Jacky went to investigate, Mr Brown was not there but Jacky found what looked like semen on a lady's cardigan and in her hair. She immediately washed the lady and her cardigan. Jacky was very concerned but didn't feel confident that she could safely raise the matter with Mr Brown. It would be a matter of her word against his.

A few weeks later, she entered a room occupied by a lady with dementia. Mr Brown seemed to have his groin in the lady's face and Jacky thought he might be forcing oral sex on her. She left the room and got a colleague. When Mr Brown had gone, they returned and, with a clean swab, took a specimen from the lady's mouth.

Jacky had the swab analysed by the forensic laboratory and it was shown to contain semen. She spoke with the police who arrested Mr Brown. He initially denied the accusation but, when confronted with the forensic evidence, pleaded guilty to two charges of indecent assault and was jailed for four years.

How would you describe the course of action that Jacky took?

Why was it necessary for her to take that course of action?

5.5.2 Know how and when to report any resource or operational difficulties that might affect the delivery of safe care

Resources are the things that an organisation needs in order to provide a service. 'Operations' is the term used to describe the ways an organisation delivers its service. Inadequate resources and operational difficulties that affect the delivery of care include:

- insufficient staff. Tight budgets often mean that organisations are understaffed and cannot afford staff cover. Not enough staff means poor standards of care

- inexperienced staff. Care work has a large turnover of staff and many people who start a career in care have little, if any, experience. Inexperienced staff also means poor standards of care
- insufficient training. Insufficient training means poor standards of care and leads to accidents and injuries
- out-dated procedures, which result in dangerous work practices
- a poor working environment, e.g. cramped, too dark, too hot. Poor working environments cause accidents and injuries
- old and poorly maintained equipment, which is dangerous and causes accidents and injuries
- security problems, e.g. unwelcome visitors, who put people's safety and well being at risk
- people who take risks, have challenging behaviour or who behave in unexpected ways, all of which threaten health and safety.

Employers of social care workers, like social care workers, have to obey a GSCC Code of Practice. The Code of Practice for Employers of Social Care

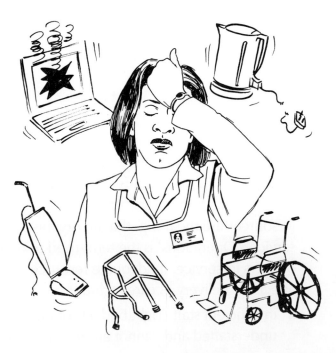

Safe care?

Workers states that your employer:

- must have procedures that allow you to report inadequate resources or operational difficulties that might affect the delivery of safe care

- must work with you to deal with problems due to inadequate resources or operational difficulties.

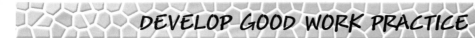

DEVELOP GOOD WORK PRACTICE 5.5.2

ACTIVITY 59

1 Identify three or four inadequate resources and/or operational difficulties that might affect the delivery of safe care at your workplace.

2 Read your organisation's procedures for reporting inadequate resources and operational difficulties, and make notes on how and when to report the ones you identified.

3 Why is it important that you report inadequate resources and operational difficulties?

5.5.3 Know how and when and your duty to report the practice of colleagues which may be unsafe

Unsafe work practices in care work include:

- not following care plans, which means people's needs are not met.
- not following procedures, perhaps because of ignorance or a lack of understanding. If care workers do not know or understand procedures, their work will not support people's right to protection from danger and harm.
- doing activities for which no training has been given. Remember, care workers are not allowed to do activities for which they have not been trained; and some skills need to be updated on a regular basis, e.g. emergency first aid
- not reporting accidents, injuries, infections, dangerous incidents and hazards such as dangerous equipment. Making reports means problems can be dealt with and prevented in the future
- discrimination, including bullying and harassment – you learnt about the effects of discrimination in Chapter 1
- abuse and neglect of people needing support, and self-neglect, e.g. working when ill or dependent on drugs and alcohol. The effects of abuse, neglect and self-neglect are described above.

As you know, you have a legal duty to follow health and safety procedures and to report hazards and unsafe practices (see Chapter 3). The Code of Practice for Employers of Social Care Workers states that your employer must:

- have procedures that allow you to report dangerous, discriminatory and abusive behaviour and practice
- deal with these reports promptly, effectively and openly.

DEVELOP GOOD WORK PRACTICE

5.5.3

ACTIVITY 60

1 Identify three or four work practices at your workplace that might be unsafe.

2 Read your organisation's procedures for reporting unsafe work practices, and make notes on how and when to report the ones you identified.

3 Why is it important that you report unsafe work practices?

5.5.4 Know what to do if you have followed your organisation's policies and procedures to report suspected abuse, neglect, operational difficulties or unsafe practices, and no action has been taken

You *must* follow your organisation's procedures when reporting:

- inadequate resources and operational difficulties that might affect the delivery of safe care at your workplace
- unsafe working practices of your colleagues.

If you are concerned that your organisation has not dealt with your reports suitably, you may 'blow the whistle'. However, to be covered by the Public Interest Disclosure Act (see above) you need to make a 'protected disclosure'. This means raising your concern as described in the guidelines set out in the Act. There are a number of ways to make a protected disclosure:

1. Talk to your manager. If this isn't an option, check whether your organisation has a procedure in place for voicing concerns and, if it has, follow it.

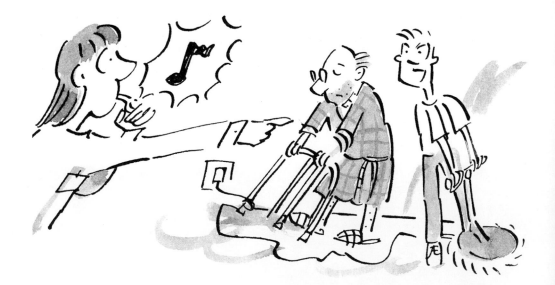

Whistle blowing

2. If the issue still hasn't been dealt with, contact the Commission for Social Care Inspection (CSCI). The role of the CSCI is to inspect and report on care services, to improve social care and to stamp out bad practice. At the time of writing (September 2006) contact details for the CSCI are: St Nicholas Building, St Nicholas Street, Newcastle upon Tyne NE1 1NB; Tel: 0191 233 3600/0845 025 0120; Fax: 0191 233 3569; www.csci.
org.uk

3. If you believe you will be treated unfairly if you go to your employer or the CSCI, or you have already raised your concern with your employer or the CSCI and no action has been taken or you have not been informed of any action, contact the media or someone in a position of authority, e.g. your local MP or the police.

CHECK YOUR UNDERSTANDING

5.5.4

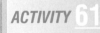

You have been asked to assist a colleague to transfer a frail, elderly lady from her bed to the bath. You notice that the hoist is long overdue a service. Your colleague says she dislikes using hoists – she says it is quicker and easier to man-handle people even though the elderly lady is obviously in pain as she drags her out of bed. Because you know that the hoist is unsafe to use, that man-handling is not allowed and that to inflict pain on someone is a form of abuse, you report the situation to your manager.

What would you do if your organisation took no action?

6 Develop as a worker

To improve the way you work, increase your chances of promotion and stay fulfilled in your job, you need to continually develop your knowledge and understanding of care work, learn new skills, stay up-to-date with care issues and look after yourself physically and emotionally. The aim of this chapter is to help you identify where to get advice, information and support to help you develop as a worker, raise your awareness of your learning needs and encourage you to take responsibility for your development. It also builds on what you have learnt about effective communication, your role as a worker and how to maintain safety at work.

Successful completion of the activities in this chapter will enable you to demonstrate your understanding of the Common Induction Standard *Develop as a worker*. It will also give you an opportunity to develop evidence for key skills unit Communication at level 1.

What is covered in this chapter?

This chapter contributes to the knowledge and understanding you need for the following NVQ Care units at level 2:
HSC 23 : Develop your knowledge and practice
HSC 24 : Ensure your own actions support the care, protection and well being of individuals

6.1 SUPPORT AND SUPERVISION

6.1.1 Know how to get advice, information and support about the organisation, your own role and responsibilities and the role/responsibilities of others

We all need advice, information and support from time to time if we are to enjoy our jobs, perform them well and be satisfied in what we do.

Sources of advice, information and support available to you about your organisation include:

- the Commission for Social Care Inspection (CSCI), which inspects and produces reports about social care providers such as care homes
- your Local Authority Social Services Department
- your organisation's Mission Statement, Care Charters and policies
- your organisation's Human Resources staff
- your colleagues and line manager
- your organisation's staff development officer, training officer and NVQ assessor
- your Trades Union representative.

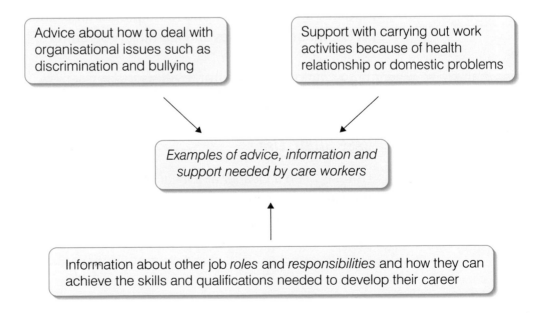

Advice about how to deal with organisational issues such as discrimination and bullying

Support with carrying out work activities because of health relationship or domestic problems

Examples of advice, information and support needed by care workers

Information about other job *roles* and *responsibilities* and how they can achieve the skills and qualifications needed to develop their career

Sources of advice, information and support available to you about your roles and responsibilities and those of other people at work include:

- job descriptions and person specifications
- contracts of employment
- your organisation's human resources staff
- the people you support and your colleagues and line manager
- your organisation's policies and procedures
- the GSCC Codes of Practice (see Chapter 2)
- the CSCI National Minimum Standards for the care setting in which you work (see Chapter 5)
- Skills for Care, which developed the Common Induction Standards qualification that this book is helping you to achieve
- your Trades Union representative
- your organisation's staff development officer, training officer and NVQ assessor
- your mentor or workplace learning representative/support worker
- social care learning programmes delivered by your Local Authority Adult Education Department and College of Further Education
- the media, e.g. specialist social care publications such as textbooks and journals; educational TV and radio programmes, training videos and DVDs; internet websites and learning programmes.

CHECK YOUR UNDERSTANDING

6.1.1

ACTIVITY 62

CASE STUDY: *Lisa*

Lisa has been a cleaner at a local school for a number of years. She's thinking about joining your organisation as a cook or a care worker. She doesn't know anything about your organisation, nor about the roles and responsibilities of a cook and care worker.

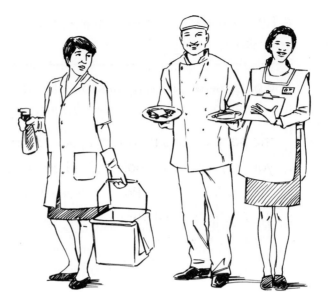

What shall I do?

Complete the table with sources of advice, information and support that you think would help Lisa make a decision about her future.

Sources of advice, information and support about your organisation	Sources of advice, information and support about the role and responsibilities of a cook	Sources of advice, information and support about the role and responsibilities of a care worker

6.1.2 Understand the purpose and arrangements for supervision in your work setting

The purpose of supervision is to make sure that good work practices are developed and maintained. Supervision is essential in organisations that provide caring services. Where it doesn't exist or is ineffective, care workers have low morale and little, if any, job satisfaction; and the quality of service to the people they support is poor.

Supervision should be carried out by workers who have been trained to do the job. The table below describes the four main purposes of supervision and how your supervisor uses these purposes to ensure that you develop and maintain good work practices.

Purpose of supervision	How your supervisor uses supervision to help you develop and maintain good work practice
1 Quality assurance	• To make sure you know and understand your roles and responsibilities • To make sure you use the Social Care Code of Practice and the principles of care in your work • To make sure you have access to resources that allow you to work safely
2 Learning and development	• To identify your learning and performance needs • To identify appropriate learning opportunities and new experiences • To encourage you to use these learning opportunities and new experiences to improve your learning and performance • To make sure you stay up-to-date with ways of working
3 Support	• To create a safe and secure environment in which you feel able to discuss how you feel about your work and the way you do it • To help you identify and manage problems such as stress that could affect your work • To identify and provide resources that will help you manage stressful situations

	• To challenge you to think in different ways about the way you work and deal with situations and relationships
4 Shared decision-making	• To plan with you the best way for you to improve your learning and performance – action plans that relate to your professional development are called Personal Development Plans (PDPs)
	• To agree your roles and responsibilities with you
	• To prevent you from doing activities for which you have no training or experience
	• To prevent you from being exposed to situations that you would find very difficult to cope with

There are two types of supervision: formal and informal.

Formal supervision happens on a planned basis and should take place in private. Appraisal is an example of formal supervision. You will be asked to attend appraisal meetings at times laid down in your organisation's policy on supervision, e.g. annually or every six months.

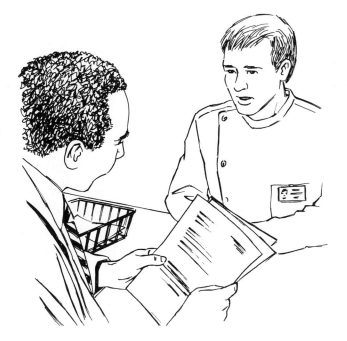

Appraisal

167

Informal supervision is on-going. It takes place 'on the job', that is, while you are working and when your knowledge and performance can be observed. Informal supervision happens all the time and takes the form of discussions with colleagues, your line manager and with learning mentors and NVQ assessors who know what you need to learn and who want you to succeed. Informal supervision also takes the form of discussions with the people you support, who are in an excellent position to monitor how you do your job!

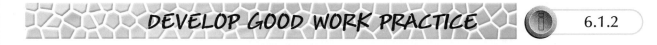

DEVELOP GOOD WORK PRACTICE — 6.1.2

ACTIVITY 63

Talk to your line manager about the purpose and arrangements for supervision at your workplace, and note down:

- why you will be supervised
- who, in addition to your line manager, will be responsible for supervising you
- how you will be supervised
- when you will be supervised.

6.1.3 Know how to use supervision effectively

For informal supervision to be effective, it is important that you have a positive attitude to criticism about the way you do your job. Welcome feedback and use it to think about what you do and to improve your performance and develop your skills. If you are not confident that you can change in the way that you have been asked, be honest about how you feel and discuss alternatives.

For formal supervision sessions to be effective, it is important to prepare beforehand. Think about and make notes on:

- the feedback people give you about the way you do your work, how well you think you perform, the skills and knowledge you need to develop and how you think you could achieve them
- any problems you have that could affect your work, e.g. domestic and relationship problems and problems related to your workload, your working environment and your work with the people you support
- ways that things could be improved. Your ideas will be welcomed if they are well thought through.

Discuss your thoughts and ideas with the person who supervises you. Listen to what they say and be open to their suggestions about how you can make changes. Again, if you are not confident that you can change in the way you have been asked, be honest about how you feel and discuss alternatives.

You should come away from a formal supervision session with an updated Personal Development Plan that records:

- your Continuing Professional Development (CPD) needs and when and how they will be met
- suggestions for how you can manage problems such as stress
- the resources you need to help you work more safely and when your line manager will put them in place
- how any operational difficulties that get in the way of safe practice are going to be dealt with by your line manager.

Following supervision, it is your responsibility to action the learning and development aspects of your CPD. You will read how you can do this shortly. It is also your responsibility to action any suggestions that were made to help you to deal with stress.

Stress can be good in small doses. It can stimulate us to work harder and deal with challenging situations, such as taking faulty goods back to a shop. But when we cannot escape from stressful circumstances, for example when we are stuck in traffic which will make us late for an appointment, when we do not get on with a colleague or someone we support, or when the bills are piling up and there is no chance of being able to pay them, stress can be very damaging to our health.

Stress affects people emotionally and physically. You need to know how to deal with stress before it affects your health. Everyone is different but the following ideas might work for you:

- do something active – stress produces energy so use it up by going for a run, doing some exercise, making a cup of tea
- tell someone how you feel – it helps to talk and get things off your chest
- do something to relax – having a bath, lighting an aromatherapy candle and practising yoga are peaceful and calming things to do.

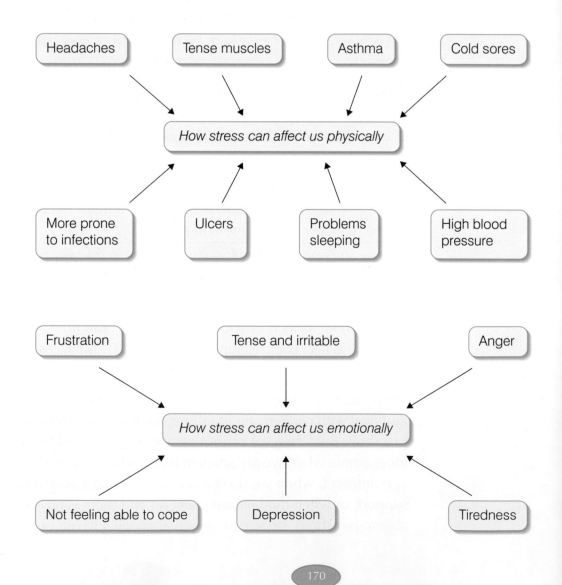

If you are stressed to the point where your health begins to suffer, you will not be able to do your job properly. In such a situation, you must talk with your line manager. They may be able to help. If not, they will be able to refer you on to someone else who can, such as your GP, therapists, counsellors, telephone help-lines and voluntary organisations who specialise in stress-related problems.

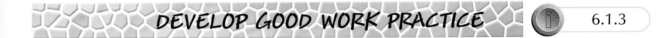

DEVELOP GOOD WORK PRACTICE　　6.1.3

ACTIVITY 64

Ask your line manager to check that you know how to use supervision effectively and to sign the Witness Statement to indicate your competence.

Witness Statement

_____ (name of worker)

understands how to use supervision effectively.

_____ (name of line manager)

_____ (signature of line manager)

_____ (date)

6.2 KNOWLEDGE AND SKILL DEVELOPMENT

6.2.1 Understand the need to gain skills and knowledge to support and develop your work

Take a few minutes to think about everything you have learned while you have been working in care. Include all the hands-on caring tasks as well as the behind-the-scenes chores like housework, answering the telephone, completing records, meetings and discussions.

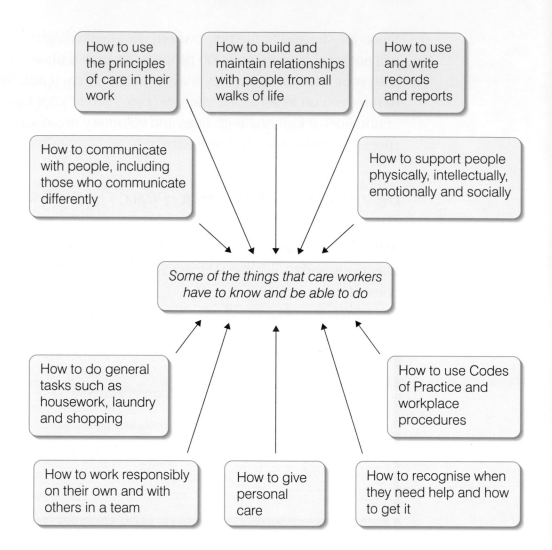

You will probably be quite surprised at how clever you are! Care work is multi-skilled and care workers need to have a wide knowledge and understanding.

The Code of Practice for Social Care workers requires that you take responsibility for maintaining and improving your knowledge and skills. We call this Continuing Professional Development (CPD) and, as you read earlier, your Personal Development Plan records your CPD needs and describes how you can meet them.

How did you develop the skills you have now? Much of what you do you will have been learnt by 'shadowing' a senior colleague, to see how they do things, and then by having a go yourself. You might have attended some in-house training sessions such as emergency first aid and moving and handling. Doing things yourself – 'hands on' learning – is a good way to develop the skills you need for your work.

Listening and reading are good ways to improve your learning. For example, when you first started work, you will have learnt about the principles of care and how to use them by listening to what your line manager told you. Your line manager will also have told you about workplace policies and procedures, the Code of Practice and the records and reports you have to use and write. And of course reading this book and doing the activities have given you the opportunity to improve and provide evidence for your learning about what makes for good care practice.

How can you continue to learn and improve your performance so that you become valued and respected by everyone you work with? The answer is to:

- ask the people you support and your colleagues for feedback on your current performance
- reflect on your own performance and think about how you need to develop.

Then, armed with feedback and your own ideas about your skills and learning needs, check out and take advantage of all the learning opportunities available to you. You could, for example:

- continue to watch and listen to your colleagues – their experience is invaluable and something you should take advantage of
- attend training sessions that your line manager or manager organises for you
- read specialist care magazines and journals – these will keep you informed about your job role and up-to-date on issues to do with caring

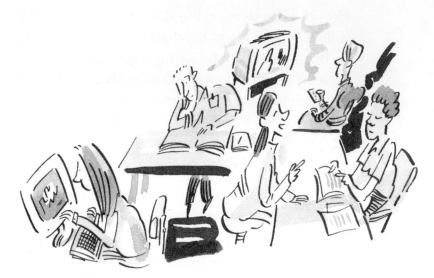

There are numerous ways to imrove your knowledge

- watch educational TV programmes, videos and DVDs
- check out care-related internet websites – these will also keep you up-to-date on a wide variety of care topics
- enrol on a course at your local school or college, for example to learn about areas of care that are quite new to you or brush up your communication skills
- enrol on a care-related internet course – the advantage of these courses is that you can study at a time that is best for you
- join a voluntary group or sports team, help run Cubs or Brownies, get together with a crowd of friends and take part in pub quizzes. Being with other people in situations like these will help you develop teamwork skills.

Don't just go for the learning opportunities that are planned for you at work. Check out opportunities for yourself, ones that you know you will enjoy. You learn more when you have fun! Apart from making you better at your job and more likely to get promotion, improving your learning will earn you respect from others and increase your self-confidence and self-esteem.

ACTIVITY 65

- Reflect on, and talk to colleagues and the people you work with about your performance at work, and make a list of the skills and areas of knowledge that you need to develop. Be honest!
- Why do you need to develop these skills and areas of knowledge?
- How can you develop these skills and areas of knowledge?

6.2.2 Know how to work with your line manager to agree and follow your personal development plan

You read earlier that one of the purposes of supervision is to agree and plan with you how you might develop your learning and skills. It is a smart idea to include **SMART** learning and skills development targets in your Personal Development Plan. **SMART** targets are:

- **S**pecific, i.e. clear and precise, so you know exactly what you are supposed to be learning and getting better at

- **M**easurable, so you can find out whether you have been successful. Certificates measure success, as does feedback from colleagues, the people you support and so on
- **A**chievable, i.e. within your capabilities. If you are asked to do something you are not capable of doing, the odds are you will not be successful
- **R**ealistic, i.e. sensible and practical. It would not be practical to ask you to do a full time course at College as well as work seven days a week!
- **T**ime-related, because it always helps to have a deadline to work to.

Make sure you agree and understand the targets in your Personal Development Plan. Talk them through with the person who is supervising you and find out who can help you to achieve them.

When you are sure that you understand what you have to do, work through your plan to achieve your targets on time. Use different ways of learning to find the ones that suit you best, e.g. learning through listening to or watching others, doing things yourself, reading, writing, discussions and so on. Make changes suggested by your supervisor to develop your skills; and use the people you support, your colleagues, line manager and so on to help you meet your targets.

Periodically review your progress and achievements by checking your Personal Development Plan. Do this with the person who supervises you, during a formal appraisal or informally, over a cup of tea when you are having a break from work. Discuss what you have learned, what skills you have developed and whether you have done what you set out to do.

Sometimes you won't achieve your targets by the deadline you set. If you don't, ask yourself why. For example, did you give yourself enough time? Did your personal life or finances prevent you from successful studying? If you don't achieve your targets by the deadline you set, be prepared to adapt them and set further deadlines. The secret is to not give up, because there are numerous benefits associated with knowledge and skill development!

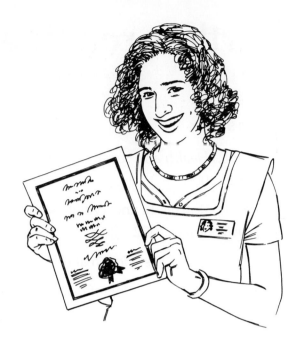

The benefits of personal development

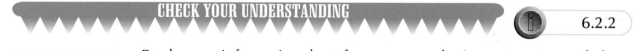

CHECK YOUR UNDERSTANDING

6.2.2

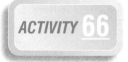

Produce an information sheet for someone who is new to care work that describes the purpose of a Personal Development Plan and how they should use it to support their knowledge and skills development.

Further reading

Textbooks

Clarke, L., *Health and Social Care for Foundation GNVQ*, 2nd edn. Nelson Thornes, 2000

Clarke, L., Rowell, K. and White, M., *An Entry Level Course in Caring*, Nelson Thornes, 2002

Michie, V., *BTEC First Health and Social Care*, Nelson Thornes, 2006

Trickett, J., *The Prevention of Food Poisoning*, Nelson Thornes, 2001

Wells, J., *The Home Care Workers Handbook*, UKHCA, 1999

Leaflets

Areas of Risk – Home Hygiene, Domestos

Avoiding Slips, Trips and Broken Hips, Department of Trade and Industry, 1999

Care Homes for Older People: National Minimum Standards Care Homes Regs, Department of Health

COSHH: The New Brief Guide for Employers, Health and Safety Executive, INDG136L

Electrical Safety Leads to Fire Safety, Home Office, FL04

Employee's Guide to the Health and Safety at Work Act, Scriptographic Publications

Essential Steps to Safe, Clean Care, Department of Health/NHS

Everyone's Guide to RIDDOR 95, Health and Safety Executive, 1995

Falls – How to Avoid Them and How to Cope, Age Concern/Royal Society for the Prevention of Accidents

Fire Kills – You Can Prevent It. Get a Plan Get Out Alive, Home Office

First Aid – Basic Advice on First Aid at Work, Health and Safety Executive

Food Safety and Temperature Control, Foodlink

Get the Balance Right, British Meat Nutrition Education Service

Getting to Grips with Manual Handling, Health and Safety Executive

A Guide to the General Food Hygiene Regulations 1995 – Food Safety, Department of Health

How to Choose and Use Fire Extinguishers for the Home, Home Office

In Doubt? Keep Them Out, Home Office

Preventing Slips, Trips and Falls at Work, Health and Safety Executive

Safe as Houses, Department of Health

A Safer Place Self-audit Tool – Combating Violence Against Social Care Staff, Department of Health, 2001

Safety and Security at Home, Age Concern England

A Short Guide to the Personal Protective Equipment at Work Regs 1992, Health and Safety Executive

So You Think You're Safe at Home? Department of Trade and Industry/ Royal Society for the Prevention of Accidents

Stay Safe at Home, Department of Trade and Industry

Step Up to Safety, Department of Trade and Industry

The Health Guide, Health Promotion England

Violence at Work, Health and Safety Executive

What to do if You're Worried a Child is Being Abused, Department of Health

Working Alone in Safety, Health and Safety Executive

Working Together to Reduce Stress at Work – A guide for employees, International Stress Management Association UK, 2004

Websites

www.gscc.org.uk – General Social Care Council

www.drc-gb.org – Disability Rights Commission

www.dh.gov.uk – Department of Health

www.niscc.info – Northern Ireland Social Care Council

www.sssc.uk.com – Scottish Social Services Council

www.ccwales.org.uk – Care Council for Wales

www.csci.org.uk – Commission for Social Care Inspection

www.alzheimers.org.uk – The Alzheimer's Society

www.hse.gov.uk – The Health and Safety Executive

www.firekills.gov.uk – Information about Fire Safety

www.nursing-standard.co.uk – Journal for nurses

www.bupa.co.uk – BUPA

www.corecharity.org.uk – Information about digestive disorders

www.sense.org.uk – UK Deafblind charity

www.deafblind.com/ – Information about Deafblindness

www.crb.gov.uk – Criminal Records Bureau

www.freedomtocare.org – Whistle blower support group

www.everychildmatters.gov.uk – Guidance on The Children Act 2004

www.careconnectlearn.co.uk – National learndirect centre for health and social care

www.dti.gov.uk – Department of Trade and Industry

www.nhs.uk – The National Health Service

www.topssengland.net – Skills for Care

www.socialcareassociation.co.uk – The Social Care Association

www.skillsforhealth.org.uk – Training Organisation for the Health Care Sector

www.hmso.gov.uk/acts/acts2000/ukpga-20000014-en.pdf – Care Standards Act

www.carestandards.org.uk – The National Care Standards Commission

www.ace.org.uk – Age Concern England

www.pcaw.co.uk – Public Concern at Work, Whistleblowing

Glossary

Accountable	Answerable, responsible.
Advocates	People who talk or act on behalf of others.
Aids and adaptations	Things that help people with their day-to-day living activities.
Asphyxiation	Suffocation.
Care package	A group of services brought together to achieve the care plan.
Care plans	A plan to provide care services to an individual (or family).
Care service providers	Organisations that provide caring services.
Care values	The beliefs that underpin care work.
Care workers	People who are employed to support people who have care needs.
Carers	People who support and care for others but who are not paid for what they do.
Catheter	A tube that is inserted into the urethra to drain urine away from the bladder.
Codes of Practice	Rules that govern ways of doing things.
Colostomy	An operation that creates an opening from the bowel to the body surface.
Commission for Social Care Inspection	The organisation that inspects providers of caring services.

Confidentiality	To do with being discreet and keeping things private.
Consent	Permission.
Cross-infection	The spread of infection from one person to another.
Discrimination	Treating people unfairly because of the way they have been labelled, stereotyped or pre-judged.
Diverse	Different, varied.
Equal opportunities	Treating everyone fairly by giving them equal access to the same opportunities in life.
Extended families	Mother, father and the children, plus other relatives who either live close by or live with them.
First language	The language someone uses from birth; the 'mother tongue'.
Foreign object	Something that isn't supposed to be there.
Fraud	Deception.
General Social Care Council	The organisation that regulates organisations which provide caring services.
Hazardous	Dangerous.
Hazards	Things that put health and safety at risk.
Individuals	The people receiving care and support.
Informed choices	Choices made with the benefit of knowledge.
Informed consent	Permission that is based on knowledge and understanding.
Interpreters	People who can explain the meaning of words and expressions that others have difficulty understanding.

Jargon	Technical language.
Job role	What a job is all about, e.g. cleaning.
Labelling	Describing people by characteristics such as their appearance or behaviour.
Media	Newspapers, books, magazines, the internet, etc.
Mobility problems	Difficulty moving around.
Nausea	Sickness, vomiting.
Non-statutory independent	Organisations that are not legally required to exist.
Nuclear families	Mother, father and the children living in one house.
NVQ	National Vocational Qualificiation.
Objects of reference	Objects that are used daily and which have an obvious meaning, e.g. a picture of a plate.
One-parent families	Parent and children living on their own.
PEG feeding	A method of feeding that involves inserting a tube through the abdomen wall into the stomach.
Prejudices	The ideas and beliefs we have about people without knowing or understanding them.
Pressure ulcers	Areas of damaged skin, e.g. bed sores.
Private organisations	Organisations that set out to make a profit.
Reconstituted families	Two people who are married or in a relationship for a second, third, etc. time, living with their children and step-children.

Responsibilities	The duties or tasks that are part of a job role, e.g. vacuuming, dusting and washing windows are the responsibilities of the person whose job role is to clean.
Same sex parent families	Two women or two men living with their children.
Secular beliefs	Non-religious beliefs.
Sensory impairment	Difficulty seeing or hearing.
Signer	Someone who translates speech into signs that can be understood by people with a hearing impairment.
Signs	The visible appearance of ill health.
Single-person households	Households where people live on their own.
Skills for Care	The organisation that regulates the education and training of social care workers
Standards	Benchmarks for good conduct and work practice.
Status	Position, importance.
Statutory organisations	Organisations that the law requires to be in place.
Stereotyping	A way of thinking about people because of the way they look or behave.
STI	Sexually transmitted infection.
Stoma	A surgically produced hole, usually in the wall of the abdomen, which allows waste material to pass away from the body.
Symptoms	The way someone feels when they are ill.

Translator   Someone who can express the meaning of words. and expressions into another language.

Voluntary   Non-profit making organisations.
organisations

Work setting   The place where work is carried out, e.g. a residential care home, a day care setting, a person's home.

Workplace risk   Checks to find out how safe the workplace is and
assessments   how to make it more safe.

Index

Page reference in italics indicate figures or tables